Epidural Anaesthesia

Epidural Anaesthesia: Images, Problems and Solutions

Dr Clive B. Collier, MD (UNSW), MRCP (UK), FRCA, FANZCA
Visiting Anaesthetist, Prince of Wales Private Hospital, Sydney, NSW, Australia

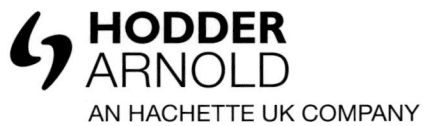
HODDER ARNOLD
AN HACHETTE UK COMPANY

First published in Great Britain in 2012 by
Hodder Arnold, an imprint of Hodder Education, a division of
Hachette UK
338 Euston Road, London NW1 3BH

http://www.hodderarnold.com

Hachette UK's policy is to use papers that are natural, renewable
and recyclable products and made from wood grown in sustainable
forests. The logging and manufacturing processes are expected to
conform to the environmental regulations of the country of origin.

Whilst the advice and information in this book are believed to
be true and accurate at the date of going to press, neither the
author[s] nor the publisher can accept any legal responsibility or
liability for any errors or omissions that may be made. In particular,
(but without limiting the generality of the preceding disclaimer)
every effort has been made to check drug dosages; however
it is still possible that errors have been missed. Furthermore,
dosage schedules are constantly being revised and new side-
effects recognized. For these reasons the reader is strongly urged
to consult the drug companies' printed instructions, and their
websites, before administering any of the drugs recommended in
this book.

British Library Cataloguing in Publication Data
A catalogue record for this book is available from the British Library

Library of Congress Cataloging-in-Publication Data
A catalog record for this book is available from the Library of
Congress

ISBN   978-1-444-15604-1

1 2 3 4 5 6 7 8 9 10

Commissioning Editor: Francesca Naish
Project Editor: Jenny Wright
Production Controller: Joanna Walker
Cover Design: Helen Townson
Index: Lisa Footitt

Typeset in 9.5/12 pt Rotis Semi Sans by Datapage
Printed and bound in Italy by Printer Trento

What do you think about this book? Or any other Hodder Arnold
title?
Please visit our website: www.hodderarnold.com

Contents

Foreword

Epidurography has been, for over three decades, the lifetime love and main body of work for Dr Clive Collier. What started, three decades ago, as an interest into the root reasons why so many major neuraxial blocks work brilliantly while others are incomplete or are outright failures has blossomed into a deep understanding of the mechanisms of regional block complications, of the nature of the subdural and intra-dural space and of the true origins of inadvertent mishaps of regional anaesthesia techniques. Dr Collier's observations, at epidurography, of the reasons for complications and the complete and partial failures (compared to some 'normal' epidurals) has produced new insights into 'the why', 'the how' and 'the when' of each of the mini-crises produced by atypical blocks.

Dr Collier's travails and the search for the truth have led to his successful MD thesis in 1994, *Some Complications of Epidural Block* and the slim but highly useful volume *An Atlas of Epidurograms: Epidural Blocks Investigated* in 1998, apart from a light-hearted, informative book for mothers-to-be entitled *Enjoy your Childbirth: The Epidural Option*. If you add to this a multitude of scientific papers, letters to the editor and a series of lectures, it is not hard to understand that Dr Collier has a wealth of experience, 'new' knowledge and expertise not available to many of us.

This new book, *Epidural Anaesthesia: Images, Problems and Solutions* has been written to redress the deficit in our knowledge base. At the time that Dr Collier penned 'the Atlas' in 1998, he had performed 100 epidurograms. Since then, he has collected just under 200 (187, to be exact) using much more sophisticated imaging techniques with much improved 3D resolution. There is no doubt that Clive Collier is the 'master of epidurography' and, thanks to his highly honed epidurogram interpretational skills, this new tome promises to be even better than the previous, outstanding offerings.

This book is a triumph, a gem and a treasure house for practising epiduralists, anaesthetists and radiologists and, possibly, for lawyers, attorneys and solicitors. While not too simplistic, it is almost a 'user handbook' covering, as it does, the overlapping spectrum of outcome variability. On the other hand, it is sufficiently comprehensive in this niche subject, the understanding of the failed block and misplaced catheter, to be seen as a reference work.

This book does presuppose that the reader has an understanding of the limits and techniques of major neuraxial blockade – epidurals, combined spinal epidurals and subarachnoid blocks – but the easy-to-read style of writing guides us skilfully through the web of intertwined and interrelated anatomical variants, pathological aberrations, spinal deformities, logistical and ergonomic deficiencies and septa in the epidural space both longitudinal and horizontal which define whether we end up with a successful block or an atypical one. We now have a reference work which complements our readings on epidural and spinal methods and techniques.

Epidurography, and Dr Collier's interpretation of his investigations, sheds much light on some of the idiosyncrasies and limitations of these techniques. The timing could not have been better. We are experiencing a revolution in regional anaesthesia. Equipment, training, drugs and safety are getting better at the same time as usage is rising. Pari passu expansion of the indications for major regional blockade in chronic pain management, palliative and supportive care, surgery, anaesthetic, perioperative medicine and diagnostics is now equalling these blocks' use in obstetric anaesthesia. Clive Collier's initial intent stems from a desire to inform our world for the sake of mothers and their infants in labour and during delivery. If this book helps one single mother it will have fulfilled its purpose. I have the sneaky feeling that it will help not only make epidurals safer for some mothers; it will give new insight to all those who perform and assist with spinal regional anaesthesia.

In the past, epidurograms have been seen as the 'playground' of the aficionado and enthusiast but I now come to see their great value in sorting out where problems lie, to anticipate potential hazards and to subsequently modify techniques. I feel that epidurography should become a routine patient care modality when a desired outcome is not achieved. This can 'inform' patient counselling and allow pre-planning for future safety and efficaciousness, enable effective medico-legal defence and satisfy intellectual and academic curiosity. This book lifts clinical experimental approaches into the realms of rational clinical applications. Post-'disaster' investigation should become a routine 'service' in much the same way that post-mortem examinations and cadaver dissection illuminated the darkness of ignorance of the structure, function and disease processes of the human body.

Epidurography is underutilized and is most utilitarian in those who present the most difficulty. Collier, in '*Images: Problems and Solutions*', teaches us how to perform the sample techniques and gain the necessary skills at interpretation. While epidurography was first described by Sicard and Forester in 1926, novel state-of-the-art imaging techniques have lifted this exercise from a restricted, limited use clinical application to a real-life re-enactment and 'repetitorium', using safe imaging media, to unravel the reasons for failure or for occurrence of complication.

I now begin to understand intimately the true anatomical nature of the epidural, subdural and intradural spaces with their compartments, tissue planes, divisions, synechiae, contents and obstructive septa which affect the spread of local anaesthetics and adjunctive medications. We now even have the images to prove them.

I congratulate Clive not only on his great reserves for descriptional artistry but for bringing to the uninitiated a deep understanding and a practical method to reach a conclusion on some of the mysteries of epidural failure and mishap.

This book is an essential read, nay, a 'look and see', for epidural 'grandmasters' and beginners (with a view to a career in obstetric and epidural anaesthesia) alike.

Stephen Gatt
President, Obstetric Anaesthesia Society of Asia and Oceania
Head of Division of Anaesthesia and Intensive Care of the Prince of Wales, Sydney
Children's and Sydney/Sydney Eye Hospital
and, previously, Prince Henry and Royal South Sydney Hospitals.
Director of Anaesthesia of the Prince of Wales Hospital and previously, Royal Hospital for Women.
Associate Professor, University of New South Wales, Sydney, Australia.

Preface

Every anaesthetist undertaking epidural blocks, whether in the fields of obstetrics, surgery or pain relief, will meet with the occasional case of complete or partial block failure and, more rarely, cases with unexplained complications, which may be life-threatening. In these situations it is surely incumbent on the individual practitioner to determine the reason for the failure or complication, rather than merely accepting a poor or uncertain outcome, with disinterest, a shrug of the shoulders, and a lame excuse to the patient. Furthermore, it is becoming increasingly likely that an individual who has suffered unnecessary pain or stress as a result of an unsatisfactory or complicated block will demand an explanation as to exactly what transpired, and the threat of medico-legal action may loom.

The technique of epidurography can usually provide the answer as to the cause of block failure or a complication. With a simple, safe, contrast injection and straightforward X-ray examination, which can be completed within 10 min even in the most basic of radiology departments, the underlying problem may, in the vast majority of cases, be clearly expounded to the reassurance of both practitioner and patient.

Epidurography has been employed in 178 cases, initially at the Royal Hospital for Women, and then at the Prince of Wales Private Hospital, in Sydney. Following a pilot study of a few successful blocks to establish the characteristics of a typical epidurogram, cases of failed or complicated blocks were kindly referred to us by our anaesthetic colleagues for investigation. The results of the first 100 studies were published in *An Atlas of Epidurograms: Epidural Blocks Investigated* (1998). In the subsequent 13 years, an additional 78 obstetric patients have been studied with epidurography. This book includes the most significant findings from the whole series, with some of the images being reproduced from the initial work, with greater clarity than previously. Our knowledge of why epidurals fail or lead to complications has advanced considerably. Particularly revealing has been the demonstration of two separate spaces in the subdural region, one previously unrecognized by anaesthetists, but now designated as the 'intradural space'. Our findings have allowed us to explain many previously baffling outcomes following atypical blocks.

Minor degrees of scoliosis, of which the patient is often unaware, seem to be a common cause of unsatisfactory epidurals in labour, especially when the current low-dose blocks are used. Our radiographs have revealed many cases of spina bifida occulta and we have attempted to demonstrate a connection with failed or complicated blocks. As our expertise and data have increased, it has become obvious that some of our previous radiographic findings had been incorrectly interpreted, and the astute reader will no doubt detect the reclassification of some images from the '*Atlas*'.

The epidurogram technique has been described in some detail, with two objectives in mind. First, in the hope that this information and our results will encourage our colleagues to undertake their own radiographic studies when faced with failed or complicated blocks, and second, to provide a reference work to assist in the interpretation of the radiographs obtained. Unfortunately, the vast majority of radiologists have little interest in epidurograms, and virtually no experience in assessing them, as the procedure is not used in current routine diagnostic practice. As a result, in the past, some of the reports on post-block epidurograms have been unreliable, regrettably even in many published cases. Consequently, it would be desirable for all regular users of epidural block to become familiar with the whole range of normal and abnormal appearances following contrast injection and epidurography.

Clive Collier
Sydney
May 2011

Acknowledgements

This study has been running for over 30 years and involved several generations of helpers, without whom little would have been achieved. I would like to thank all those individuals, many now working elsewhere or retired, who allowed me to undertake and complete this work, and make it such an enjoyable experience. A keen supporter has been Associate Professor Stephen Gatt, OAM, Chair of Division of Anaesthesia, Prince of Wales Hospital, in Sydney, who encouraged me throughout the project. Many anaesthetic colleagues offered invaluable help, but thanks are especially due to Alec Harris, Jan Lehm, Leo Lacy and Arthur Vartis, as well as countless other anaesthetic consultants and registrars.

The early epidurogram studies were undertaken in the Department of Medical Imaging at the Royal Hospital for Women, first at Paddington and then at Randwick, Sydney, by kind permission of Dr Peter Warren. The radiography staff were always most accommodating and helpful, but special thanks must go to Annette Collet, who was always happy to accede to my requests for yet another 'urgent' epidurogram, and almost invariably produced images of the highest quality with fairly basic equipment. Later epidurogram studies were undertaken at Prince of Wales Private Hospital, thanks to the services of Wales Imaging initially, and then Imaging Diagnostics Australia and Southern Radiology. At the start, my mentors and guides in relation to the medical imaging techniques and the interpretation of the results were Dr Enn Tohver, formerly Neuroradiologist at Prince of Wales Hospital, and Dr Michael Houang, Radiologist at Sydney CT and MR, who gave most freely of their time and wisdom.

Dr Nir Hoftman at the University of California Los Angeles Medical Center, USA, kindly assisted me, using his extensive knowledge of the subdural space and thoracic epidurals, and provided me with many useful images and ideas.

The obstetricians and gynaecologists involved were most understanding and cooperative throughout this work, as were the nursing staff and midwives in the operating theatres, labour and postnatal wards of the two hospitals.

I am very grateful to Professor Miguel Angel Reina (Madrid, Spain), for his excellent cooperation and invaluable advice over many years, resulting in several joint publications. He also allowed me access to his large and unique collection of electron microscopy images and diagrams. The work on the subdural and intradural spaces would not have progressed without him. Thanks also to Bruce Creevey of Kinetic Rituals (Queensland, Australia) for his expertise in constructing the models of the epidural space and dura–arachnoid interface, which have greatly clarified many of our findings, and enthralled viewers around the world. The publishing process was very smooth, pleasant and efficient thanks to the efforts of Francesca Naish and Jenny Wright at Hodder Arnold in London.

I thank Portex (Smith's Industries, Ashford, Kent, UK Ltd) and especially Cedric Russell, for their interest and friendly cooperation in the early days of this work. Finally, this project would not have been possible without the assistance of the many patients who agreed to undergo epidurography, involving, in most cases, the daunting experience of reclining on a hard, cold, X-ray table, soon after childbirth. Thank you ladies!

CHAPTER 1
INTRODUCTION: WHY INVESTIGATE ATYPICAL EPIDURAL BLOCKS?

1.1 The history of epidurography

Sicard and Forestier introduced epidurography in 1926 as an X-ray diagnostic method using Lipiodol (Fig. 1.1) and they later developed myelography.[1] Early attempts by anaesthetists to correlate the physical spread of solutions in the epidural space with the extent of the observed nerve block met with only limited success, due largely to the highly viscous nature of the contrast used. In 1940, Odom used

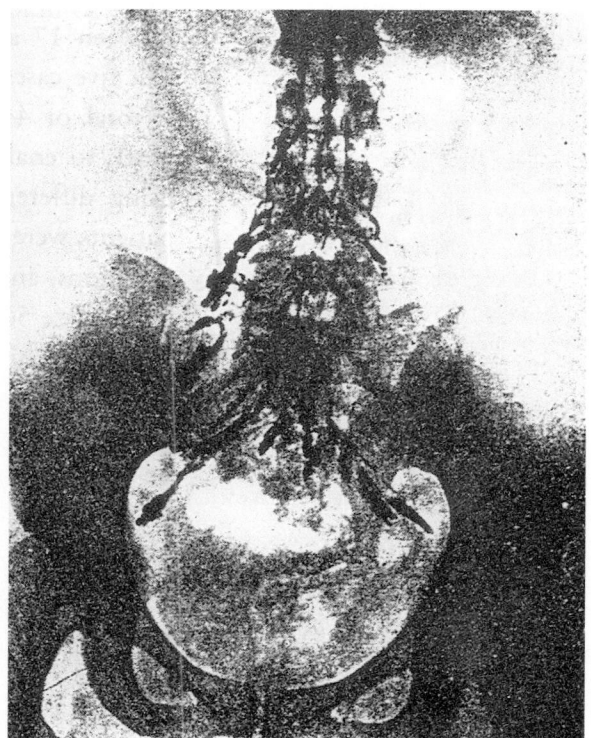

● **Fig. 1.1** One of the first epidurograms ever performed (1926), using oily contrast. The film was taken 1 h post-injection.

Lipiodol mixed with procaine in the epidural space and found that his initial X-rays showed only longitudinal spread of contrast, but films at 15–30 min, coinciding with the onset of block, showed lateral flow through the intervertebral foramina.[2] He concluded that the epidural site of action was the spinal nerves in the paravertebral space. It was not until 1954 that Bromage, using a similar technique, was able to demonstrate satisfactory nerve block in the absence of transforaminal flow.[3]

In 1959, Nishimura et al. injected epidural lignocaine (lidocaine) mixed with radioactive iodine 131 and traced the spread with a scintillation counter, mostly in a cephalad direction.[4] The segmental spread of analgesia approximately corresponded to the spread of radiation. In 1968, Shanks reported similar findings based on epidurograms in four patients who had developed unilateral block, and concluded that the spread of the radio-opaque dye meglumine iothalamate (Conray) did not necessarily mirror the spread of the local anaesthetic solution and the resulting nerve block.[5] Shanks, however, employed only very small (3 mL) volumes of the dense contrast, which were insufficient to satisfactorily demonstrate epidural spread. Many recent studies on the flow of epidural dye have also used small-volume contrast injections (3–5 mL), which often do not allow for accurate extrapolation of the precise distribution of the full volume of local anaesthetic solution that would have been used clinically (i.e. approximately 10–20 mL).

In 1973, Burn et al. reported on epidurograms in 56 patients; they found that the volume of epidural solution and the site of its injection were the most relevant factors in its distribution.[6] The rate of contrast injection and the age, height and posture of the patient had little relevance. In the same year the first generation of non-ionic water-soluble contrast media became available in the form of metrizamide (Amipaque), and correlation between epidurogram and extent of nerve-block could now be made with some confidence in individual patients. However, even today with our current contrast media the exact segmental distribution of a block cannot always be reliably predicted from an epidurogram.

1.2 Patient selection

The data in this book have been accumulated over the past 30 years, and we have performed 178 thoracolumbar epidurograms in 173 individual patients, involving 146 obstetric, 27 gynaecological and 5 general surgical cases, aged between 17 and 81 years (Fig. 1.2). Ethics committee approval was received prior to the commencement of this study, and written informed consent obtained for the first 90 studies. After that, with the technique being well established, only verbal consent was requested. All patients happily agreed to have their case histories recorded, and a few also consented to having their clinical photographs published. Only a handful of patients declined to participate in this study, with the majority of individuals being very interested in learning why their epidural had 'gone wrong', and wanting some reassurance that it would not happen again. Only three patients with iodine allergy were judged unsuitable for investigation.

A total of 46 patients, including 14 obstetric patients, were recruited following satisfactory epidural block to enable us to build up a profile of the normal epidurogram using different types and gauges of epidural catheter. A group of 32 obstetric patients was studied following blocks that had developed major complications, sometimes with block failure. Another 100 obstetric patients were investigated following inadequate blocks. In almost all of these 132 cases of atypical blocks, epidurography clearly revealed the nature and extent of the underlying problem, and advanced our knowledge of the spread of epidural, subdural and intradural injections. The majority of the abnormal obstetric blocks (78) were detected in labour, with the remainder (54) arising at caesarean section, in both elective and emergency cases.

The obstetric population is a particularly valuable group to study, as both failure and complication rates are far higher than in other fields of practice. This would seem to be principally caused by the venous congestion in the epidural space in term pregnancy, but hormonal effects appear to play a part.[7] Also of importance is the fact that the quality of the epidural block is subject to far more stringent testing in the awake obstetric patient, particularly in those undergoing caesarean section, than in her general surgical counterpart who is usually asleep or sedated. In our teaching hospital labour ward up to 7% of epidurals are classified as unsatisfactory following the initial catheter dose, although the figure drops to approximately 2% following adjustment of the catheter position and further dosing. This small group of patients with persistent unsatisfactory blocks was investigated, where possible, with epidurography.

1.3 Management of failed blocks

When all adjustments, such as change of patient position and withdrawal of the epidural catheter by 1–2 cm, together with additional doses of local anaesthetic, had failed to overcome an unsatisfactory block, our usual procedure, before the start of this study, was to remove the first epidural catheter and insert a second, usually in an adjacent interspace, although a subarachnoid block was occasionally used. We then started to request that our colleagues leave the first catheter *in situ* for later investigation. There have been no problems associated with this practice, despite the commonly expressed fears that passage of the second epidural needle might damage the first catheter, or that two epidural catheters might become knotted together.

Although it is often found following a unilateral block that the tips of both catheters are displaced laterally to the same side by a septum, or other cause, occasionally the catheter tips are located on either side of a septum and injection through both is required for satisfactory block to develop. In this situation, two catheters are essential for adequate block rather than just for diagnostic purposes.

1.4 Indications for epidurography

There would appear to be five principal indications for epidurography following a neuraxial block:

1 Diagnosis of an atypical block
2 Verification of catheter tip position

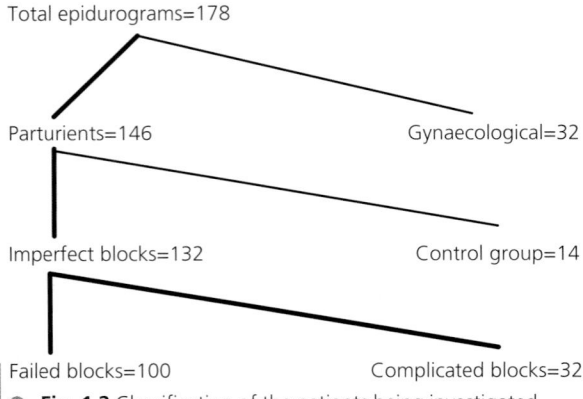

Total epidurograms=178

Parturients=146   Gynaecological=32

Imperfect blocks=132   Control group=14

Failed blocks=100   Complicated blocks=32

Fig. 1.2 Classification of the patients being investigated.

3 Definition of epidural adhesions

4 Assessment of the design and function of epidural catheters

5 Departmental research or audit into the efficiency of blocks

Radiologists have no use for epidurography in their routine practice, and even as far back as 1987 a major textbook stated that it was a method 'no longer advocated for neuroradiological diagnosis',[8] but for those studying the spread of attempted epidural block it is an invaluable tool. However, because most contemporary radiologists have no experience of epidurograms, their reporting may be unreliable, with some of these erroneous reports even appearing in published work.

1.4.1 Diagnosis of an atypical block

Emphasizing the use of epidurograms to diagnose a complicated or failed epidural block is the main objective of this book, although other workers find different roles for epidurography. The epidural complications that may be diagnosed in this way are: (1) high epidural block, (2) accidental subarachnoid block, (3) subdural block and (4) intradural block. Intravascular injection may be very difficult to demonstrate. These complicated blocks occur either alone, involving one compartment, or in combination as a multicompartment block, and may be difficult to diagnose clinically. Table 1.1 shows the incidence of these complications that developed in 32 of our obstetric patients.

Intravascular injection may be very difficult to demonstrate. The many and varied causes of block failure that we detected are listed in Table 1.2. They are usually associated with malposition of the catheter tip, with or without an anatomical anomaly, as discussed in subsequent chapters. The anatomical anomalies include septal barriers, bony deformities and fibrous adhesions.

● **Table 1.1** Classification of complicated epidural blocks in 32 obstetric patients

BLOCK	n	%
High epidural block (above T2)	13	41
Intradural block	10	31
Subarachnoid block	5	16
Subdural block	3	9
Intravascular injection	1	3

● **Table 1.2** Analysis of 100 cases of failed epidural block in obstetric patients. The most likely cause of failure is listed

CAUSE OF FAILURE	n
A septum (midline or transverse)	51
Scoliosis	23
Transforaminal escape	13
Retrograde flow	4
Expelled catheter	4
Lateral catheter tip	2
Paravertebral catheter	1
Faulty catheter	1
Adhesions post-laminectomy	1

1.4.2 Verification of catheter tip position

Knowledge of the precise position of the catheter tip may be of importance in several situations, although the use of a radio-opaque catheter may obviate the need for a contrast injection. However, some radio-opaque catheters are less pliable than their standard counterparts and more prone to breakage, reducing their usefulness.[9]

In certain groups of surgical patients, including neonates, epidurography has been advocated preoperatively to confirm the catheter position.[10] Some clinicians even site their catheters the day before major surgery.[11] Postoperatively, epidurography may be used to indicate the position of the catheter tip when attempting to correct a poorly functioning infusion, particularly when alternative forms of analgesia are unsuitable. On two occasions we have used epidurography to verify catheter position when a post-partum patient on a short-term infusion was noted to have copious volumes of clear fluid emanating from the epidural puncture site. A normal epidurogram convinced staff that the problem was not leakage of cerebrospinal fluid or epidural solution, but simply the escape of tissue oedema in a recumbent patient, and the infusion was continued.

Demonstration of the position of the catheter tip and patency of the eyes may be valuable in the management of chronic pain. Initially, following catheter insertion, the tip location may need to be ascertained, and later, in the event of block failure, repeat epidurography may reveal the nature of the problem if catheter migration or fibrosis around the tip has occurred.

1.4.3 Definition of epidural adhesions

The use of selective catheter epidurography to demonstrate fibrous adhesions in chronic pain patients, particularly following disc disease and spinal surgery, has been well described by Racz and colleagues.[12] Having defined the nature and extent of adhesions, remedial treatment with epidural lysis may be undertaken. Previously, the epidural catheters were usually directed through the sacral hiatus rather than a lumbar interspace, but with the current range of narrower and more manoeuvrable catheters the lumbar percutaneous approach appears to be proving more effective.[13]

1.4.4 Assessment of the design and function of epidural catheters

We have used epidurograms to study the direction followed by the catheter tips on insertion, as well as the pattern of flow of epidural contrast, as part of the process of assessing new epidural catheters manufactured from different materials, with varied eye configurations and gauges, prior to market release. Two particular designs were found to be unsatisfactory and abandoned. The congested epidural venous system of pregnancy appears to impede the spread of epidural solutions, and new catheters should be tested in both term-pregnant and non-pregnant subjects.

1.4.5 Departmental research or audit into the efficiency of blocks

Quality assurance audits of a departmental epidural service may be greatly assisted by knowledge of why blocks have not progressed as anticipated, and ongoing research should help to improve the efficiency and safety of the procedure. Occasionally, the results of epidurography may be helpful in medico-legal situations, when the cause of a complicated or failed block has become the subject of heated conjecture.

1.5 Arguments against epidurography

There are many detractors regarding the safety and usefulness of epidurography but most of their arguments can be soundly rebuffed. For example, there are claims that the technique is potentially dangerous with muscle spasms and epilepsy being particular problems.[14] However, such comments are outdated and refer to the subarachnoid injection of the older and long-discarded oily contrast agents

such as Myodil. Current contrast media are very safe, when iodine-allergic patients are excluded, with a low incidence of side-effects even when injection of large doses into the subarachnoid space has occurred.

Another complaint is that epidurography is, in most cases, a retrospective study and of no therapeutic value to the individual patient. While this is true in some cases, it may not apply to the obstetric patient who has endured an unsatisfactory block for labour or caesarean delivery, is considering returning for future childbirth and is requesting reassurance about further blocks. If an anatomical cause has been visualized radiologically, as is often the case, the patient can be informed and an alternative epidural or subarachnoid approach planned for the next occasion.

One cause for concern about epidurography has been expressed by Wedel, regarding the potential dangers, including subdural abscess, meningitis and even cauda equina syndrome, resulting from leaving misplaced (possibly subarachnoid) catheters in place for an unduly long period of time, such as overnight, while waiting for the radiology department to become available.[15] Such concerns appear to be considerably exaggerated and without foundation, although it would seem prudent to investigate cases of suspected subarachnoid placement within a matter of hours, rather than after a lengthy delay, although the retention of accidentally placed subarachnoid catheters for up to 24 h has been recommended in the attempted prevention of post dural puncture headache.[16] Accidental subarachnoid catheter placement is, hopefully, a rare finding and the diagnosis will usually, but not always, be made clinically apparent with the aspiration of cerebrospinal fluid (CSF), although a multicompartment block may be overlooked.

One valid criticism of post-block epidurography is that the epidural catheter associated with the problem may have been replaced, or moved from its original position prior to investigation, producing an unreliable result. In practice this does not seem to present a problem, except on the rare occasions when the catheter has either been accidentally pulled out completely or withdrawn into the subcutaneous tissues prior to contrast injection. Adequate fixation of catheters to the skin and gentle patient handling should help to dispel this problem, but we have consistently found that where there is obstruction to the free flow of epidural solutions, back-pressure results in fluid leakage around the catheter and retrograde flow to the skin. This can soak the surrounding dressings and fixation devices and may encourage catheter extrusion.

Finally, there are several authors who claim to be able to reliably diagnose epidural complications or failures on purely clinical grounds, without resorting to X-rays. This belief appears to be frequently misguided, although it is often expressed in published articles.[17,18] Examples are seen in numerous erroneous reports of unconfirmed 'atypical accidental subarachnoid blocks' that have appeared over recent years. The clinical descriptions supplied have often matched those of radiologically proven subdural block, rather than subarachnoid block as claimed.

1.6 X-Ray, CT or MRI epidurography?

The early work presented in this book was undertaken in a free-standing obstetric hospital without computed tomography (CT) or magnetic resonance imaging (MRI) facilities. Most patients were unwilling to travel to another hospital for screening, so only three patients were investigated with CT scans and two volunteers with MRI, but N. Hoftman (University of California Los Angeles Medical Center, CA, USA) has kindly provided some high-quality CT scans on three of his patients. The relatively unsophisticated use of X-rays did fulfil our requirements for a simple, rapid and inexpensive diagnostic method, and provided highly satisfactory results in most cases. Simple radiography is the method of choice as the relevant areas of the spine may be clearly visualized in two radiographic plates, rather than the multiple, more detailed sections of the CT scan, which may be difficult for anaesthetists to interpret.

If radiographic screening is available it is of great advantage for the anaesthetist involved to personally perform the contrast injection and observe the pattern of flow in 'real time', feel any possible resistance to injection and note if any patient discomfort develops. Computed tomography scans may be invaluable in the investigation of complex cases of multicompartment block (such as epidural/subdural or intradural/subarachnoid injection), as the compartments are often impossible to distinguish with X-rays. However, for routine investigation using epidurography, a CT scan is unnecessary, rather extravagant and associated with higher levels of ionizing radiation.

The role of MRI in studies of the epidural space is yet to be determined, although an increasing number of interesting reports are appearing in the literature.[19-22] (Some scans are included in chapter 3.) One advantage of MRI over the other diagnostic techniques is that it can be non-invasive, as contrast injection is not always required to display the epidural space. The epidural fat and associated blood vessels generate their own images, and most types of epidural catheter may be clearly displayed without contrast.[23]

1.7 Conclusions

We believe that there is a place for X-ray epidurography in the practice of every clinician performing epidural block, to help explain their own sporadic incidence of unusual results and to improve or modify their techniques, while advancing their knowledge and that of their colleagues. This should lead to increased patient satisfaction and decreased morbidity. Epidurography has allowed us to discover the main causes of block failure, as well as developing our awareness of complications, particularly those involving the subdural and intradural spaces.

REFERENCES

1 Sicard JA, Forestier J (1926) Roentgenologic exploration of the central nervous system with iodized oil (lipiodol). *Archives of Neurology and Psychiatry*; 16:420–434.

2 Odom CB (1940) Epidural anaesthesia in resume and prospect. *Anesthesia and Analgesia*; 19:106–112.

3 Bromage PR (1954) *Spinal Epidural Analgesia*. E & S Livingstone, Edinburgh, pp 75–83.

4 Nishimura N, Kitahara K, Kusakabe T (1959) The spread of lidocaine and I-131 solution in the epidural space. *Anesthesiology*; 20:785–788.

5 Shanks CA (1968) Four cases of unilateral epidural analgesia. *British Journal of Anaesthesia*; 40:999–1002.

6 Burn GM, Guyer PB, Langdon L (1973) The spread of solutions injected into the epidural space. A study of epidurograms in patients with the lumbosciatic syndrome. *British Journal of Anaesthesia*; 45:338–344.

7 Go KG, Blankenstein MA, Vroom TM et al. (1997) Progesterone receptors in arachnoid cysts. An immunocytochemical study in 2 cases. *Acta Neurochirurgica*; 139:349–354.

8 Kendall BE (1987) Neuroradiology of the spine. In, *A Textbook of Radiology and Imaging*; editor Sutton D. Churchill Livingstone, London pp 1484–1486.

9 Hutchison GL (1987) The severance of epidural catheters. *Anaesthesia*; 42:182–185.

10 van Niekerk J, Bax-Vermeire BMJ, Geurts JWM, Kramer PPG (1990) Epidurography in premature infants. *Anaesthesia*; 45:722–725.

11 Seeling W, Tomczak R, Merk J, Mrakovcić N (1995) Comparison of conventional and computed tomographic epidurography with contrast medium using thoracic epidural catheters. *Anaesthetist*; 44:24–36.

12 Racz JB, Heavner JE, Diede JH (1996) Lysis of epidural adhesions utilizing the epidural approach. In, *Interventional Pain Management*; editors, Waldman SD, Winnie AP. WB Saunders, Philadelphia, pp 339–351.

13 Manchikanti L, Singh V, Cash KA, Pampati V, Datta S (2009) A comparative effectiveness evaluation of percutaneous adhesiolysis and epidural steroid injections in managing lumbar post surgery syndrome: a randomized, equivalence controlled trial. *Pain Physician*; 6:E355–368.

14 Bell GT, Taylor JC (1994) Subdural block, further points. *Anaesthesia*; 49:794–795.

15 Wedel DJ (1993) Complications of regional and local anaesthesia. *Current Opinion in Anaesthesiology*; 6:830–834.

16 Dennehy KC, Rosaeg OP (1998) Intrathecal catheter insertion during labour reduces the risk of post-dural puncture headache. *Canadian Journal of Anaesthesia*; 45:42–45.

17 Harrington BE, Schmitt AM (2009) Meningeal (postdural) puncture headache, unintentional dural puncture, and the epidural blood patch: a national survey of United States practice. *Regional Anesthesia and Pain Medicine*; 34:430–437.

18 Parke TJ (1995) Variable presentation of subdural block. *Anaesthesia*; 50:177.

19 Foster PN, Stickle BR, Griffiths JO (1995) Variable presentation of subdural block. *Anaesthesia*; 50:178.

20 Westbrook JL, Renowden SA, Carrie LES (1993) Study of the extradural region using magnetic resonance imaging. *British Journal of Anaesthesia*; 71:495–498.

21 Hirabayashi JL, Shimizu R, Fukuda H, Saitoh K, Igarashi T (1996) Soft tissue anatomy within the vertebral canal in pregnant women. *British Journal of Anaesthesia*; 77:153–156.

22 Capogna G, Celleno D, Simonetti C et al. (1997) Anatomy of the lumbar epidural region using magnetic resonance imaging: a study of dimensions and a comparison of two postures. *International Journal of Obstetric Anesthesia*; 6:97–100.

23 Ralph CJ, Williams MP (1996) Subdural or epidural? Confirmation with magnetic resonance imaging. *Anaesthesia*; 51:175–177.

CHAPTER 2
THE TECHNIQUE OF EPIDUROGRAPHY

The performance of epidurography is safe, simple, inexpensive and quick, being completed within 5–10 min, with minimal discomfort to the patient.

2.1 Preparation

Before commencing, the whole procedure should be thoroughly explained to the patient and consent sought. It should be recognized that fatal reactions have been associated, on very rare occasions, with the intravascular and intrathecal use of water-soluble contrast media, and are attributed to allergic, idiosyncratic or chemical effects. Contrast injection into the epidural, subdural, intradural and subarachnoid spaces, or intravenously, appears to be free of complications, provided that patients with known iodine allergy (and thyrotoxicosis) are excluded and atopic individuals treated cautiously. Resuscitation drugs and equipment, as well as trained staff, should be readily available. Contrast injections through catheters are usually painless, but on rare occasions may produce slight transient discomfort in the back or legs. More marked pain may be experienced after subdural or intradural injection; in this case the procedure should be halted, at least temporarily.

Aspiration through the epidural catheter for blood or cerebrospinal fluid (CSF) should be attempted before injection, after removal of a filter (if present). This may reveal a misplaced catheter in the subarachnoid space, although it is not a reliable test. A small volume of contrast is usually sufficient to confirm the position of an intravascular or intrathecal catheter, but the use of larger volumes outside the epidural space should not cause undue concern, as such doses are routine in radiological practice. Most of the complications reported after intrathecal contrast injection by radiologists appear to arise from the dural puncture procedure itself, rather than the contrast. The low dose of ionizing radiation to which the patient is exposed may be a worry to a few individuals who may withhold consent, but the vast majority are undaunted.

One concern about the use of any contrast medium in lactating women is the possibility of excretion of the material in breast milk, with transfer to the neonate. Most manufacturers do not recommend the use of contrast media in nursing mothers, unless alternative arrangements can be made for feeding. However, Nielsen *et al.* demonstrated only a slow and very small transfer of metrizoate and iohexol from plasma to breast milk.[1] This is almost certainly a common finding with all high molecular weight contrast media of low lipid solubility, and there would appear to be no risk to the newborn.

The value of the investigation, either to the individual patient should they present for repeat block or for the benefit of the community in general, should be stressed. Using this approach, we have found that very few patients decline to undergo epidurography, and most enjoy viewing a previously unseen part of their anatomy.

2.2 Timing

Epidurography should be performed at the earliest convenient time postoperatively or post-delivery, as already discussed. With post-caesarean patients investigation is usually delayed for a few hours until the patient is out of bed and walking. Epidural bolus doses or infusions of local anaesthetic or opioid may be administered for pain relief in the interim, although the quality of the epidurogram is slightly diminished by the presence of other recently administered epidural solutions, with blurring of the contrast outline (see, for example, Fig. 3.7, p.15). After the epidurogram, continuing analgesia by bolus or infusion appears to be unaffected by the presence of residual contrast.

2.3 Equipment

The highest quality results are achieved if the investigation is performed in the radiology department, but portable X-ray equipment may give a satisfactory picture at the bedside if patient transfer is difficult or unsuitable and particularly if only catheter tip location is required.

Even the most modestly equipped radiology department is sufficient for epidurography, as only straightforward anteroposterior and lateral plates of the thoracolumbar spine are required for a basic study. Fluoroscopic screening with videotape, disc or DVD recording adds more detailed information and allows later review, but is not essential as in most cases it is gross changes that are being sought and these are usually clearly identifiable on standard X-ray films. However, the presence of obstructive septa or multicompartment blocks may be missed on 'still' films and only revealed with moving images.

In the radiology department we have successfully used a Bucky table with screening initially in the supine and then in the left lateral position, and occasionally in an oblique plane, with exposure of one or two plates at each location. The use of a C-arm image intensifier, when available, is preferred, as turning of the patient, which is often a painful manoeuvre in postsurgical patients, is avoided. If screening is used, the operator should adopt appropriate safety measures including a protective leaded apron, neck shield, glasses and leaded gloves, although the gloves make injection of contrast a rather cumbersome procedure.

The risk to the patient of radiation exposure is difficult to estimate but appears to be minimal with modern low-dose pulsed fluoroscopy. Typical figures for radiation levels would appear to be 0.01 mSv for a single exposure, which is less than the naturally occurring background radiation in 1 day.[2] If three exposures are made, the radiation is expected to be less than 0.05 mSv.[2]

2.4 The contrast medium

The contrast medium used should be safe if injected into the epidural space, but safe also should accidental injection occur into a vein or the subarachnoid space. We initially used metrizamide (Amipaque) as the contrast medium, but better results were obtained when the tri-iodinated non-ionic water soluble medium iohexol (Omnipaque) became available. This was later replaced by iotrolan (Isovist) and currently iopamidol (Isovue). The manufacturer's (Bracco Diagnostics Inc, Princeton, NJ, USA) package insert, dated September 2006, for iopamidol states that it is recommended for intrathecal use,[3] an opinion supported by the current edition of MIMS (Australia, 2009)[4] although the US FDA in March 2007 stated that iopamidol is 'not for intrathecal use'.[5] Instead, Bracco recommend Isovue-M, an iopamidol solution with either 200 mg/mL or 300 mg/mL of iodine for intrathecal use, even though these agents appear to contain identical components to the standard Isovue solutions.[6]

The more concentrated iopamidol solution containing 300 mg/mL produced a far more distinct image in the epidural space than the weaker dose of 240 mg/mL which was initially available to us, and was preferred for routine use. The bottles of contrast were stored in a warming cabinet to reduce the viscosity of the solution before injection.

A standard contrast dose of 10–13 mL (depending on patient size) was initially chosen as we wished to compare the extent of filling of the epidural space between individuals. However, in later cases the injected volume was determined by the adequacy of filling of the space, as assessed on screening, and doses up to 20 mL were occasionally given with improved results. The selected dose was injected over 1–3 min with the patient in the supine position and the epidural filter removed, as this presents a considerable resistance to flow. If the patient complained of any pain or discomfort, the injection was halted, at least temporarily.

2.5 Side-effects

No major side-effects have resulted from the contrast injection in our 178 cases. Ten patients complained of transient pain on injection. The first developed moderate bilateral discomfort involving the anterior thighs (L3) during her contrast injection, which was revealed to be subarachnoid, while the second complained of a mild burning sensation in her back during epidural injection. Five patients with intradural injections also complained of transient back or leg pain.

In all 10 patients who reported pain, injection was halted until symptoms subsided and then resumed more slowly. This proved satisfactory in six patients, but pain recurred in four patients (three with intradural injection) and the procedure was abandoned without any sequelae. There were no other complications.

2.6 Results

The patients were shown their X-ray films or videotapes/discs or DVDs as soon as they became available, and the findings were discussed. Most individuals showed considerable fascination when the results were revealed and explained. A letter describing any unusual findings, together with suggestions for the management of future blocks was forwarded to the patient and their attending doctor, with a copy filed in their hospital records. The X-rays also provided useful information for discussion at departmental morbidity and audit meetings. Three-dimensional modelling of a few of the epidurograms was undertaken, based on anteroposterior (AP), lateral and oblique radiographs, using 3D Studio Max (Autodesk Inc, San Rafeal, CA, USA). The resulting still images appear throughout the book, and the moving-images may be visualized on the web-site that accompanies this book or at http://www.epidural.net.au.

REFERENCES

1 Nielsen ST, Matheson I, Rasmussen JN et al. (1987) Excretion of iohexol and metrizoate in human breast milk. *Acta Radiologica Scandinavica*; 5:523–526.

2 Taenzer AH, Clark CV, Kovarik WD (2010) Experience with 724 epidurograms for epidural catheter placement in pediatric anesthesia. *Regional Anesthesia and Pain Medicine*; 35:432–435.

3 Bracco Diagnostics Inc. (2006) *Product Information: Isovue* (Package Insert, revised 28 September 2006). Bracco Diagnostics Inc., Princeton, NJ, USA.

4 MIMS (2009) *MIMS (Australia) Annual*. UBM Medica Pty Ltd, St Leonards.

5 FDA (2007) *Isovue – Iopamidol injection* (Revised March 2007), official PDF. FDA, Silver Spring, MD, USA. Available at: at http://www.fda.gov (accessed 10/6/2011).

6 Bracco Diagnostics Inc. (2001) *Isovue-M Material Safety Data Sheet*. Bracco Diagnostics Inc., Princeton, NJ, USA.

CHAPTER 3
THE TYPICAL EPIDUROGRAM

A 'typical' epidurogram profile was compiled from the X-ray findings following clinically satisfactory blocks in 46 subjects, comprising 32 gynaecological patients and 14 parturients. Although there was considerable variation, depending on the gauge and design of the particular epidural catheter in use and the age of the patient, with the elderly often showing some rather bizarre appearances, a few characteristic features became evident.

The typical epidurogram appearance in young and middle-aged adults, using a slightly rigid 17-gauge (g)nylon catheter (Portex Ltd, Ashford, Kent, UK) with a closed end and three lateral eyes spaced at 8, 12 and 16 mm from the tip, are described below. The catheters were inserted by anaesthetists of all grades and experience, to a depth of 3–6 cm within the epidural space, following loss-of-resistance testing with air, in the majority of cases, with the remainder having loss-of-resistance to saline (or occasionally local anaesthetic). Where the catheter tip was clearly seen on X-ray, its path has been highlighted in red, or occasionally blue, if more than one catheter was present. The vast majority of the catheters were directed cephalad through an upward-pointing Tuohy needle bevel, and most continued in this direction (see page 127).

3.1 Epidurogram findings following satisfactory block

3.1.1 Anteroposterior view

In the anteroposterior view (AP; Fig. 3.1a), injection of 10–13 mL of contrast is seen to produce the classical 'Christmas-tree appearance' with the 'tree-trunk' spread over approximately eight or nine vertebral levels, typically six or seven vertebral segments cephalad of the catheter tip and one or two caudal to it. In the example shown (Fig. 3.1a), which also appears as a three-dimensional model (Fig. 3.1b), contrast spread covered 13 segments. In another patient (Fig. 3.2a) 12 segments were involved. In both of these cases, contrast ascended as high as T4, although neither patient

had developed a sensory block above T9, following the injection of 20 mL 0.25% bupivacaine.

The characteristic appearance of the 'tree-trunk' is that of a body of contrast usually much denser in its lateral aspects than in the midline. The lateral columns are not of consistent width, usually being wider at the level of the intervertebral discs and narrowing at the level of the vertebral pedicles. The 'branches of the tree' are composed of contrast spreading around the spinal nerves, and then emerging through the intervertebral foramina and running laterally for a variable distance. In the lower thoracic and upper lumbar spine the diameter of the epidural space is relatively wide reflecting the underlying lumbar enlargement of the cord, and the spinal nerves curve obliquely downwards as they emerge from the subarachnoid space (Fig. 3.1a). In the upper thoracic region, the cord is narrower and the smaller spinal nerves exit the cord almost horizontally, so that the spread of contrast tends to be less prominent and at 90° to the axis of the cord (Fig. 3.2b). The lower lumbar and sacral nerves run almost vertically downwards from the spinal cord and the spread of contrast reflects this (Figs 3.3 and 3.4).

3.1.2 Contrast flow through intervertebral foramina

Typically, some contrast escaped through the intervertebral foramina at most of the vertebral levels which showed an accompanying central body of contrast, and the presence of such escape did appear to correlate well with an adequate segmental block at that level, when appropriate doses of epidural local anaesthetic had been administered.

The contrast escape (or 'spill') was usually fairly symmetrical bilaterally, but occasionally was predominantly at the level of one particular spinal nerve, or pair of nerves, and demonstrated marked and distant spread of contrast at this level, as appeared through the left T12–L1 intervertebral foramen in Fig. 3.1a and b, and through the right L3–4 in Fig. 3.3. Occasionally, in this series, contrast was seen to emerge through sacral foramina (Fig. 3.4), although others have reported this as a frequent finding.[1]

Contrast escaping through the intervertebral foramina usually followed the direction of flow within the vertebral

● **Fig. 3.1** (a) Typical AP (anteroposterior) epidurogram with 'Christmas tree' appearance from T11 to L5. The transforaminal escape of contrast at several vertebral levels is indicated by the red arrows, with only a single outline appearing at some, and a double outline at others. In this case, there is a large volume of contrast spill through the left T12–L1 intervertebral foramen. (b) Three-dimensional model of the epidural space, in the same patient. AP view. 'Contrast' escaping from the left T12–L1 intervertebral foramen is prominent.

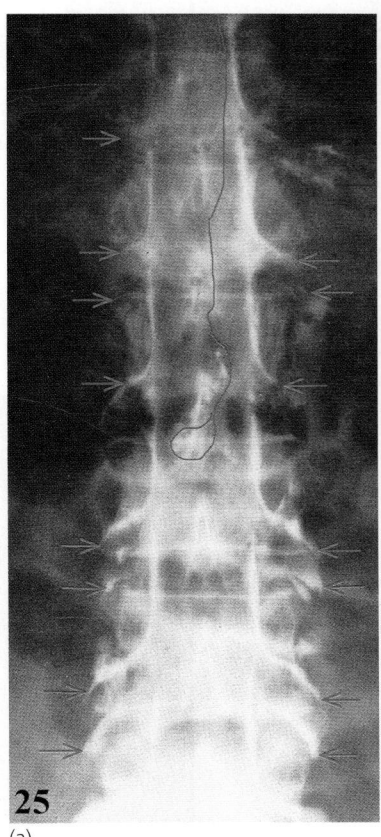

(a)

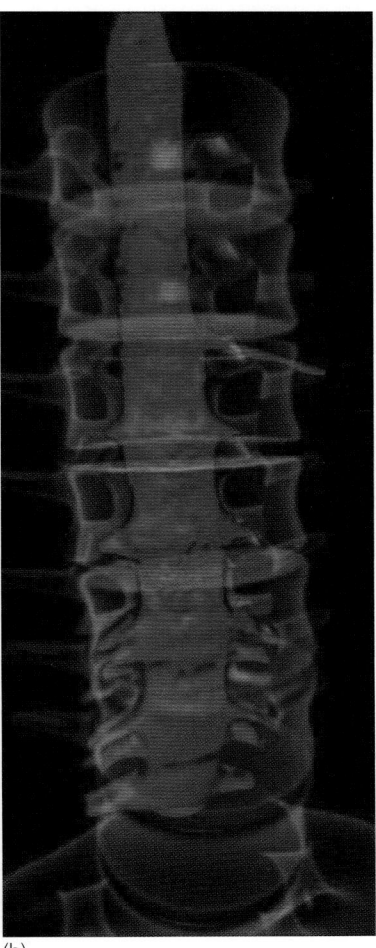

(b)

canal, as would be expected, with upper thoracic contrast continuing horizontally, lower thoracic and upper lumbar flowing diagonally downwards, and lower lumbar and sacral flow running almost vertically downwards. Exceptions were seen in some elderly patients where cephalad spread of escaping contrast was occasionally seen (see, for example, Fig. 3.10a, p.21).

3.1.3 Air bubbles

A few bubbles of air in the epidural space are a fairly constant feature of epidurograms (Fig. 3.3), as noted by Hogan in all 20 patients he studied with computed tomography (CT) scan,[2] and they represent either air remaining from the loss of resistance test during epidural needle insertion, air sucked into the epidural space following puncture of the ligamentum flavum, or possibly air accidentally contained in infusion tubing and syringes. Where repeated attempts at epidural insertion have been made, the accumulation of an

increased volume of air bubbles is expected (see, for example, Fig. 7.7a, p.93). However, we could not relate the presence of excessive air bubbles to the prior failure of a block, as have some other workers.[2-4]

3.1.4 Lateral view

In the lateral view, the marked anterior (or ventral) and posterior (or dorsal) layers of contrast are usually a standard feature (Figs 3.5 and 3.6). The anterior layer lies between the dural sac and the anterior wall of the spinal canal and is frequently of greater density than the posterior layer. The width of the anterior layer may not be uniform, as behind an intervertebral disc it tends to be narrow, with enlargement behind the centre of the vertebral body. The distance between the anterior layer and the posterior aspect of the vertebral bodies cannot be used as a diagnostic criterion to distinguish epidural from subdural contrast, as the apparent thickness of the epidural fat and connective tissue varies considerably

● **Fig. 3.2** (a) Typical AP (anteroposterior) epidurogram with 'Christmas tree' appearance from T5 to L4, and transforaminal contrast spill at most levels. The left-sided escape of thoracic contrast from T6 to T9 is arrowed. (b) A more detailed AP epidurogram in the same patient, highlighting the thoracic spread of contrast. The left T6–T9 spinal nerves are arrowed.

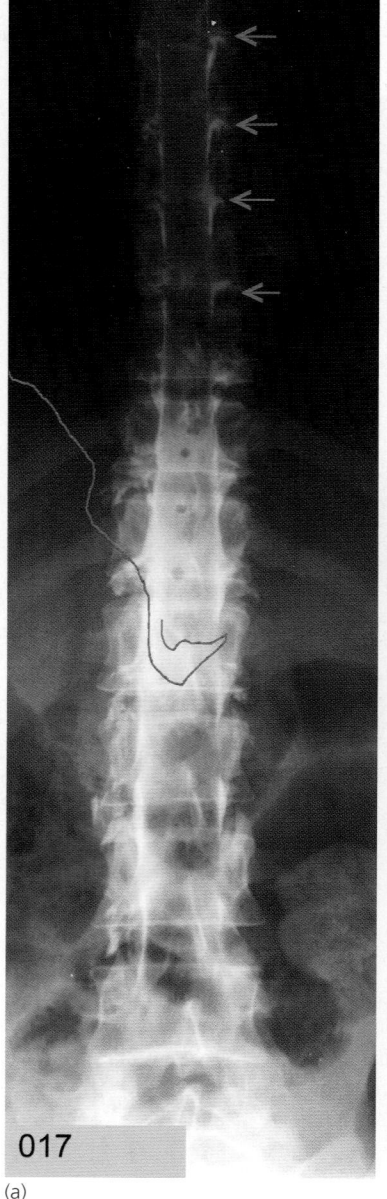

(a)

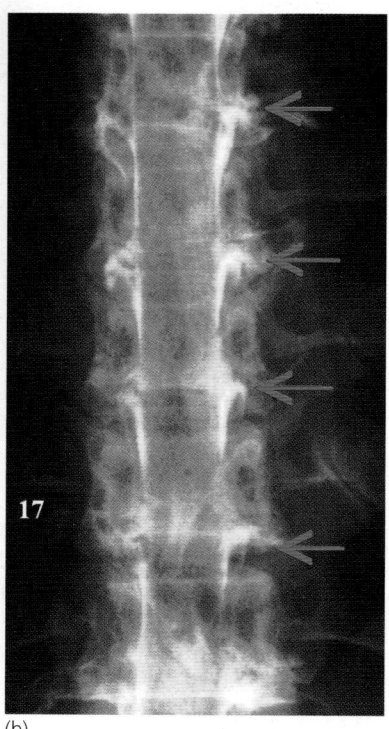

(b)

between patients (and even in the same patient with varying amounts of contrast material). There is some disagreement about whether the anterior epidural space exists above the mid-thoracic level. It is generally agreed that the dura and the posterior longitudinal ligament are fused in this area,[5] but Hogan has claimed the fusion is only intermittent.[6] In our current work, contrast filling of the anterior space in the upper thoracic spine was seen, but only rarely.

The posterior contrast band tends to be wider than the anterior with a less radio-opaque mid-zone between the two, surrounding the intervertebral foramina with their nerve-roots, blood vessels and areolar tissue usually outlined by contrast (Fig. 3.5, blue arrows). The posterior band usually extends a little more cephalad than the anterior, but in some cases, particularly where kyphosis is present in elderly patients, the difference may be marked, as seen in Fig. 3.11b (p.22) where the posterior column extended up to T4, with the anterior only up to T10. All the lateral radiographs in this work were taken in the left lateral position.

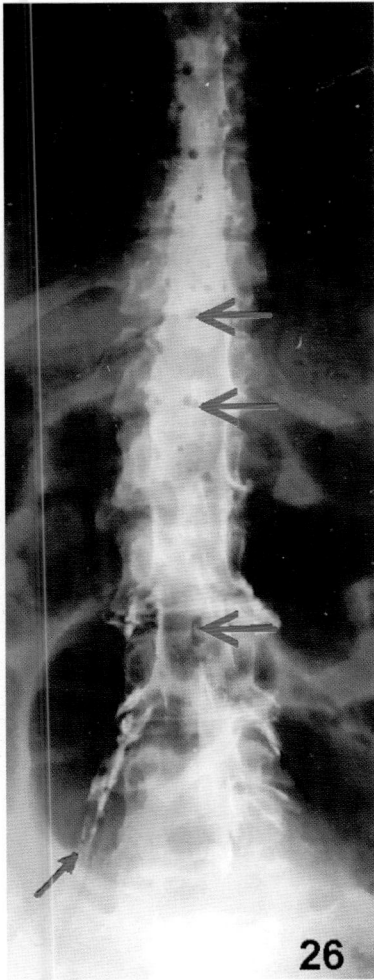

26

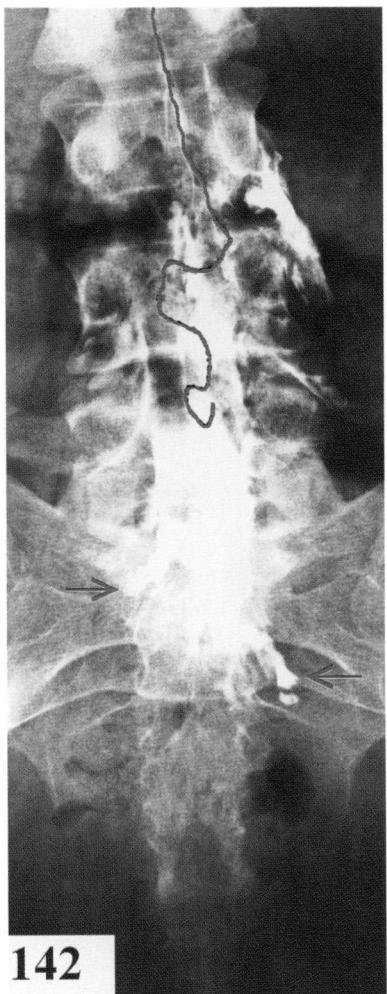

142

● **Fig. 3.3** Fairly typical anteroposterior (AP) epidurogram showing marked contrast escape from the right L3–4 intervertebral foramen (lower arrow). Multiple small air bubbles are present within the body of epidural contrast (upper arrows).

● **Fig. 3.4** Anteroposterior (AP) epidurogram following L4–5 epidural insertion, showing a low body of contrast from L3 downwards, with marked contrast escape from the left S2 and right S1 foramina (arrowed).

3.1.5 Prior epidural fluid administration

The presence of fluid in the epidural space before contrast injection may alter the resulting images. As already mentioned, the prior administration of local anaesthetic or opioid, by bolus or infusion, produces a blurred, flocculent outline to the body of contrast (Fig. 3.7, arrowed), although interpretation of the resulting picture, which in this case shows a right unilateral contrast spread with a presumed midline septum, is barely impeded. The leakage of a large volume of cerebrospinal fluid into the epidural space, following accidental dural puncture, may, however, obstruct the flow of contrast, as described later (see Figs 4.8 and 4.9, pp.36–37).

3.2 Fluoroscopic screening findings

On screening the AP epidurogram after lumbar epidural contrast injection the gradual development of the appearances already described becomes apparent. The pattern of flow of epidural contrast is best appreciated by viewing the videotape/DVD recordings on the accompanying web-site but in their absence a series of still images will give some concept of the real-time appearances. One of two different sequences of contrast spread usually emerges, depending largely on the situation of the catheter tip, the type of catheter and the presence of obstructive septa, or

13

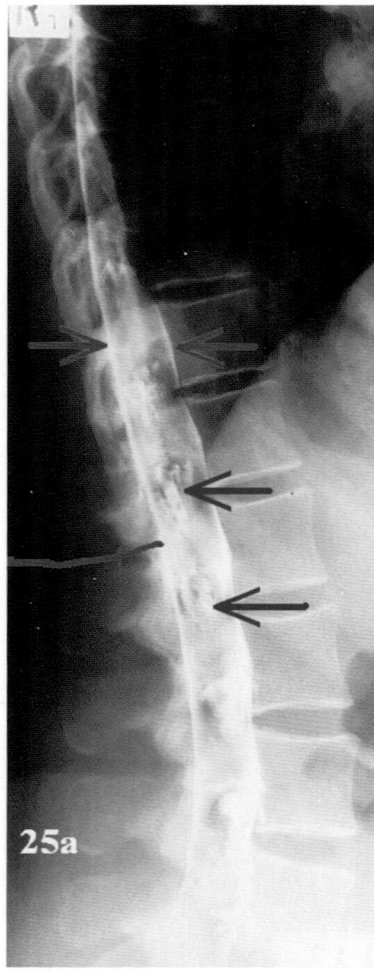

● **Fig. 3.5** Lateral epidurogram showing typical contrast distribution from T8 to L5. The anterior and posterior columns are arrowed in red, and the L1–2, L2–3 intervertebral foramina in blue. (Same patient as Fig. 3.1, p.11.)

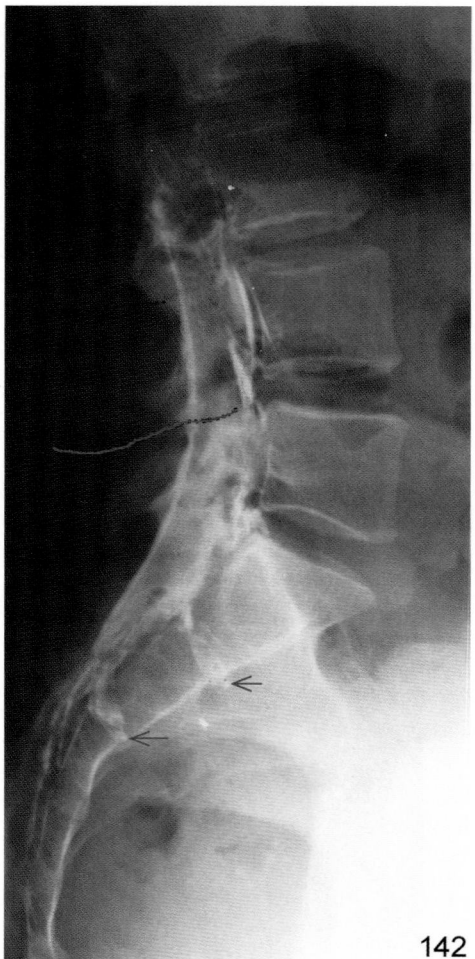

● **Fig. 3.6** Lateral epidurogram showing low lumbosacral contrast distribution, below L3. Contrast escaping from the S1 and S2 sacral foramina is arrowed. (Same patient as Fig. 3.4, p.13.)

bony abnormality in the epidural space (see later). The most common initial appearance is the spread of contrast in lateral channels, usually bilateral. Less commonly a central aggregation of contrast is the first feature. Examples of these sequences will now be described.

3.2.1 Lateral channelling of contrast

The most common pattern of images is shown in Fig. 3.8a–c, with approximately 3–4 mL of contrast injected over 15–20 s between each image. The distinguishing feature is the early filling (within 15 s) of the lateral bands or channels of contrast (red arrows) up to T8 on the left, and T12 on the right

(Fig. 3.8a). Only after 40 s does the central body of contrast start to appear (Fig. 3.8b), accompanied by transforaminal spill (blue arrows). After 60 s the mass of contrast shows thickening and consolidation (Fig. 3.8c), with increased spill, which is more clearly seen in the corresponding radiograph (Fig. 3.8d), with contrast extending from T7 to L5. The clinical findings were of satisfactory analgesia for labour, but poor sacral block for forceps delivery, despite the extensive contrast spread.

In this case the lateral channelling of contrast was similar on left and right. Unilateral channelling, or predominance of one particular side, is seen more frequently when the catheter tip is placed laterally, or a septal barrier impedes flow.

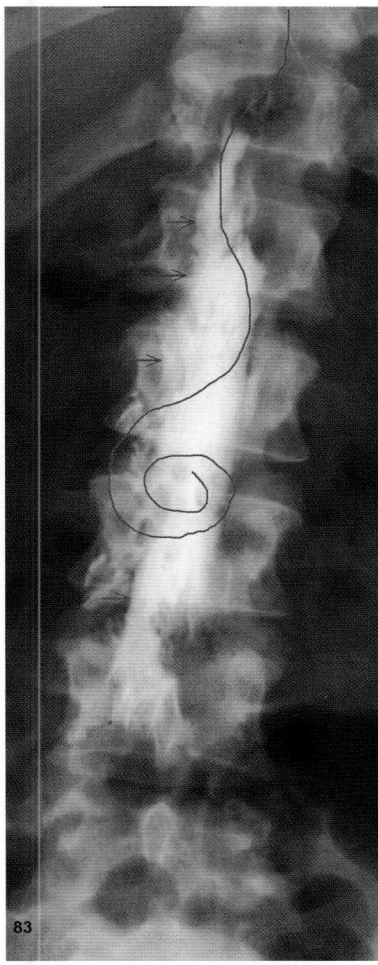

● **Fig. 3.7** Anteroposterior (AP) epidurogram after patient-controlled epidural analgesia (PCEA) infusion for several hours. The right border of the contrast is blurred (arrows) by the presence of fluid. The contrast is almost entirely right-sided because of a midline septum.

3.2.2 Central aggregation of contrast

The other common pattern of contrast flow is now described, with the catheter tip, in this case, positioned near the midline at L4–5. The initial contrast flow appears, after 20 s, as a narrow, dense central aggregation that flows fairly rapidly, in a cephalad direction, with only a slow and small caudal extension (Fig. 3.9a). The left L4–5 nerve spill is evident (blue arrow). With continuing injection, the central mass of contrast thickens and ascends to L3 by 30 s, and lateral channelling commences (Fig. 3.9b). After 50 s,

bilateral lateral columns are evident, with thickening of the mass of central contrast and increasing transforaminal spill (Fig. 3.9c). Further consolidation of the entire mass of contrast occurs up until 70 s (Fig. 3.9d). Views of the corresponding radiographs are shown for comparison in Fig. 3.9e and f. The spread of contrast is seen to be patchy with the lateral columns being slightly attenuated. The clinical findings were of satisfactory analgesia for labour and delivery.

3.3 Epidurograms in older patients

Although most of the work in this study was undertaken in parturients, a few older gynaecological patients were also investigated. In patients over 60 years of age, or those below this age with a degenerative disease of the spine, an unusual epidurogram picture often emerged. Early workers in the field of epidurography considered there was decreased lateral flow of contrast in the elderly, with higher vertical spread, consequent on fibrotic and bony changes, which reduced the patency of the intervertebral foramina.[7] Others attributed the increased cephalad spread to arteriosclerosis, decreased neural population and increased compliance in the epidural space. More recent research using the epiduroscope has shown that the fatty tissue in the epidural space diminishes with age, and the space becomes more widely patent.[7] Whatever the cause, increased cephalad spread of both local anaesthetics and contrast material is frequently seen in this group of patients. The relationship between high spread and the kyphoscoliosis commonly seen in the aged patient is described in Chapter 8.

3.3.1 Epidurogram findings in two older patients after satisfactory block

Figure 3.10a (p. 21) shows the epidurogram following an uneventful epidural block in an 86-year-old gynaecological patient, where a terminal eye catheter had been inserted at L3–4. Marked bony degenerative changes are evident, as well as patchy spread of contrast between T11 and L4, with lateral and central pools of contrast and very extensive foraminal spill. While most of the spill is directed caudally with a downward curve as usual, the L1 root spill on the left is extensive (arrowed) and is directed cephalad, which is rather unusual. The lateral epidurogram (Fig. 3.10b) confirms the presence of kyphosis with contrast extending right across the epidural space,

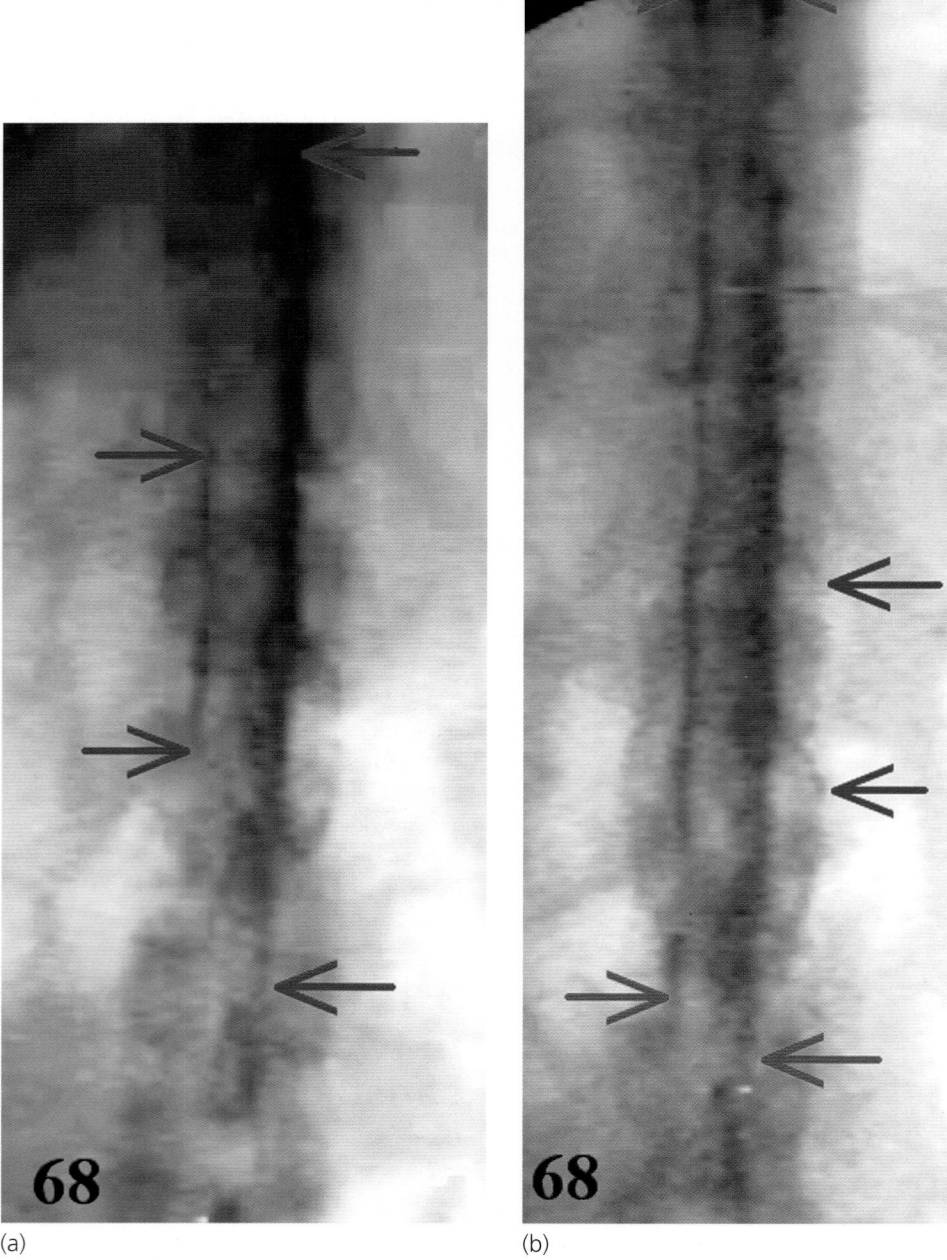

● **Fig. 3.8** (a–c) Sequence of anteroposterior (AP) fluoroscopic images during contrast injection. (a) At 15 s post-injection, there is bilateral channelling of contrast from T8 to L4 on the left and from T12 to L2 on the right (red arrows). (b) By 40 s, contrast has spread to T8 bilaterally (red arrows), with early central filling. Left L1–2 and L3–4 transforaminal spill is appearing (blue arrows).

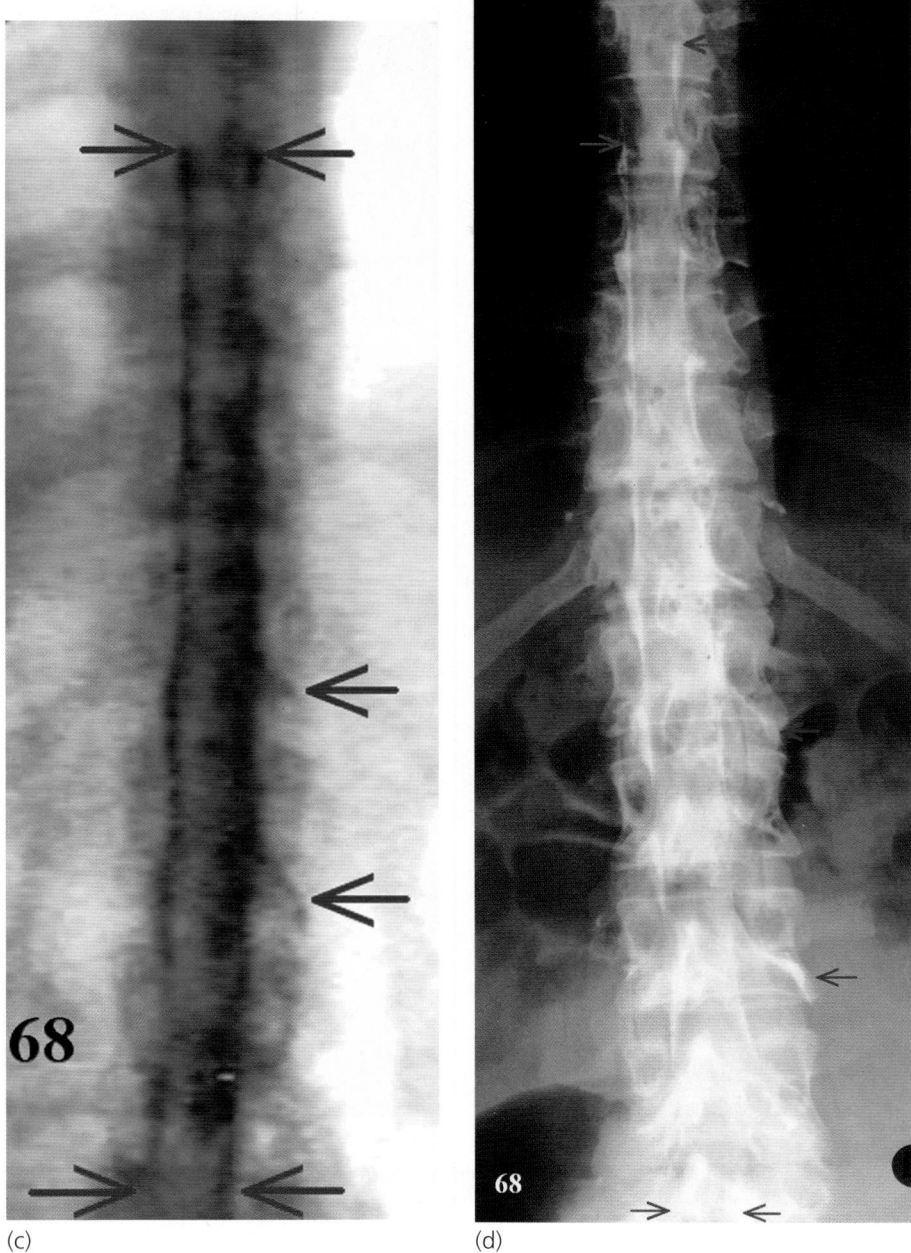

(c)   (d)

● **Fig. 3.8** (Continued) (c) Around 60 s, the central body of contrast has become more dense. The left L1–2 and L3–4 transforaminal spill is more pronounced. (d) An AP radiograph, in the same patient, at 70 s, showing extensive bilateral contrast spread from T7 to L5 (red arrows) and prominent spill at left L1–2 and L3–4 (blue arrows).

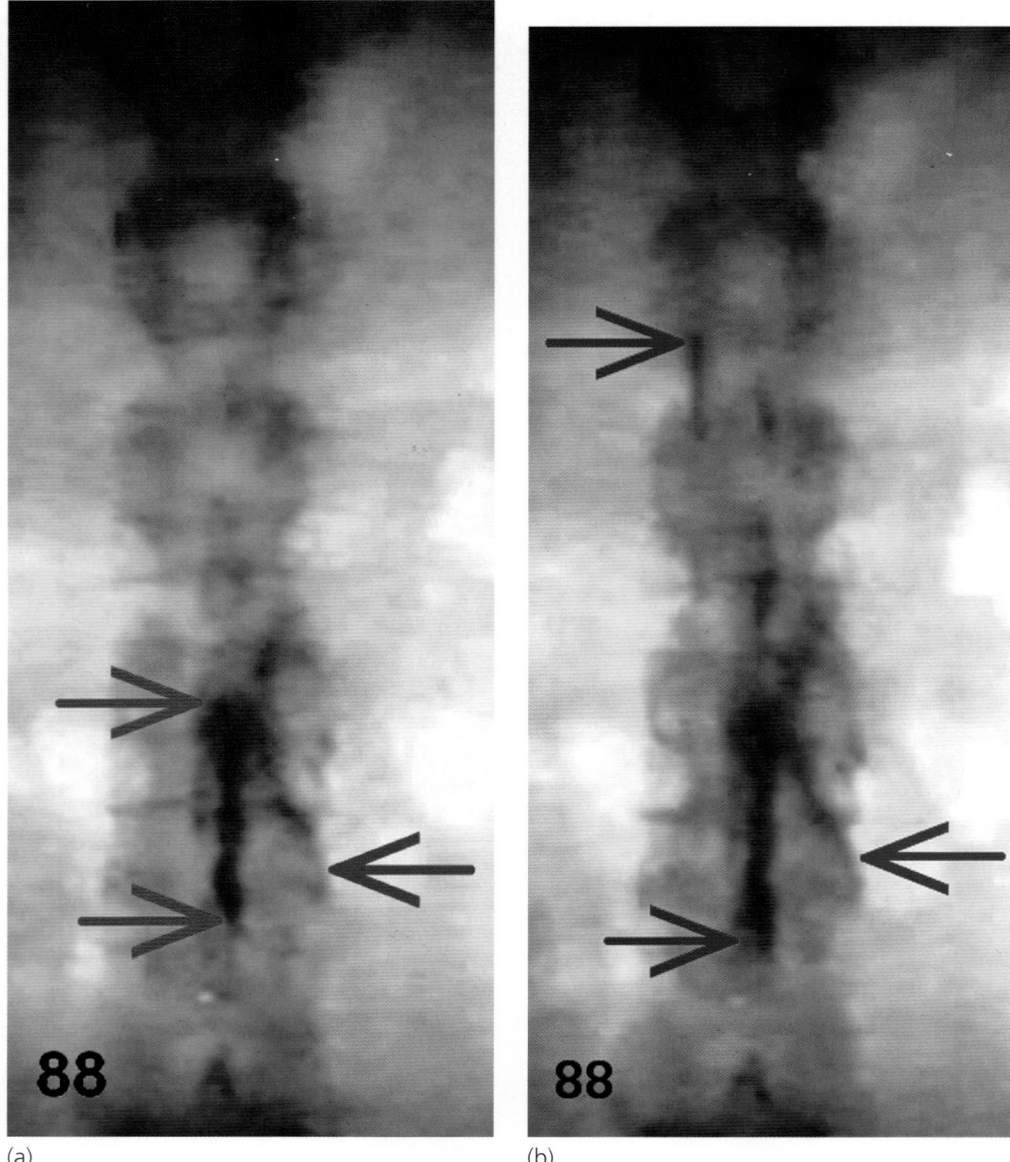

(a)   (b)

Fig. 3.9 (a–d) Sequence of anteroposterior (AP) fluoroscopic images during contrast injection. (a) At 20 s, a small central body of contrast appears (red arrows), with spill through the left L4–5 intervertebral foramen (blue arrow). (b) By 30 s, the central body of contrast has widened and spread to L3 (lower red arrow), and lateral spread of contrast has appeared up to L2 on the right (upper red arrow). There is increased left L4–5 transforaminal nerve spill (blue arrow).

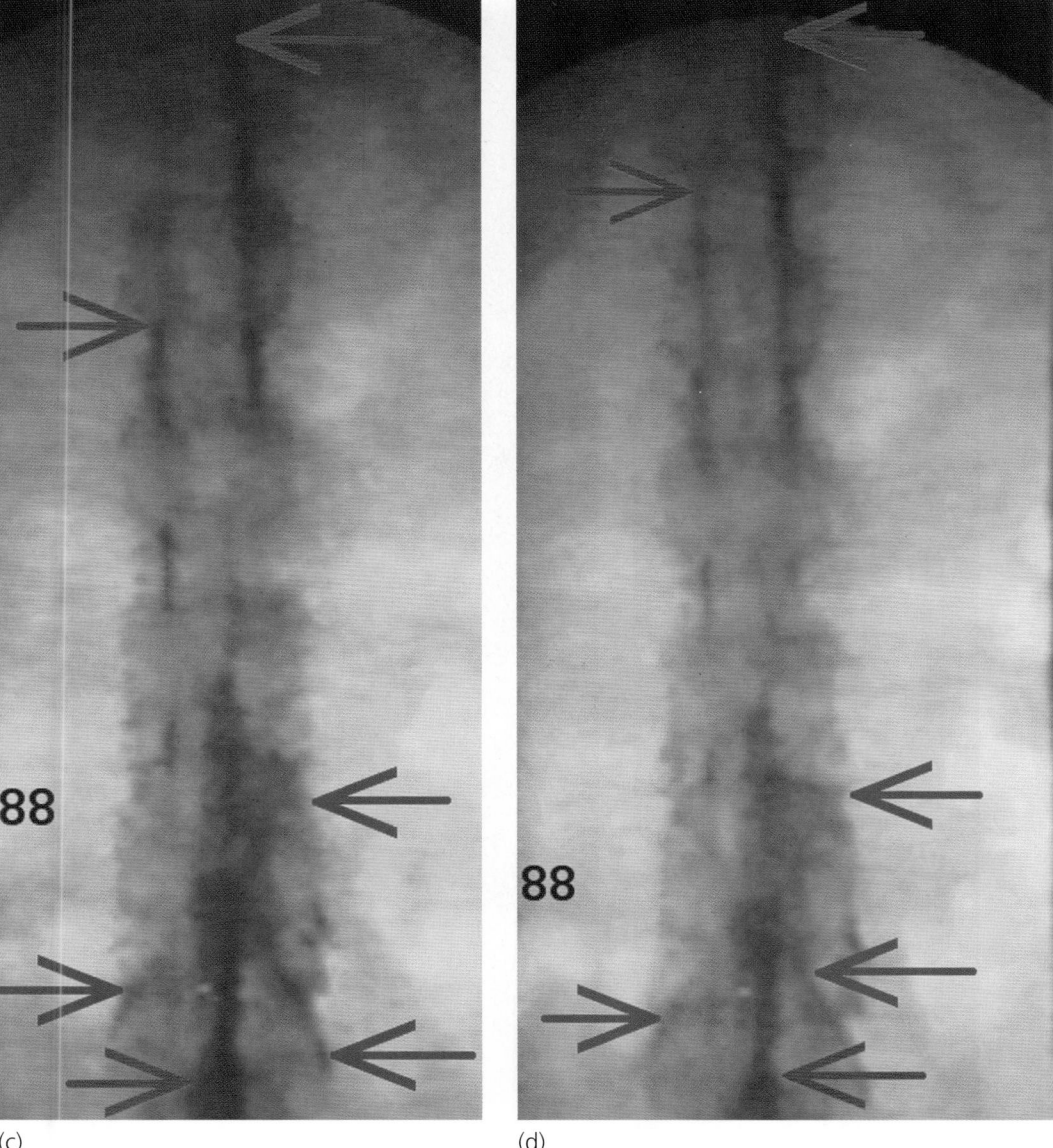

(c)   (d)

Fig. 3.9 (Continued) (c) After 50 s, the central body of contrast has again extended, while lateral spread has reached L1 on the left and T10 on the right (red arrows). The left L3–4 transforaminal spill has become more prominent and right L4–5 spill has appeared (blue arrows). (d) At 70 s, the contrast has extended to left T12 and generally thickened in appearance.

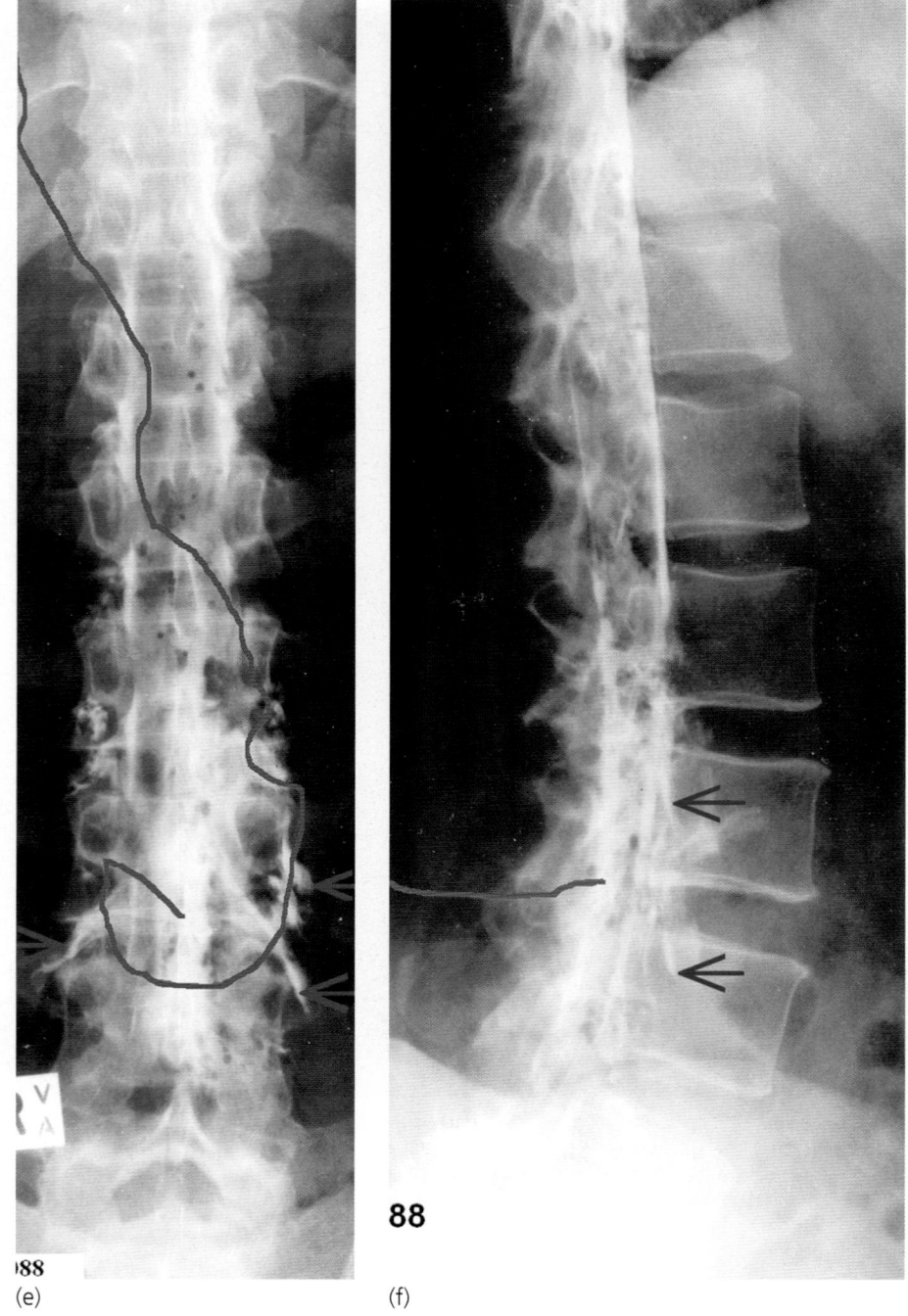

(e)   (f)

● **Fig. 3.9** (Continued) (e) The AP radiograph, in the same patient at 80 s, shows the asymmetrical central body of contrast and the lateral channelling, which is a little patchy. The L3–4 and L4–5 transforaminal spill is arrowed in blue. (f) The lateral radiograph at 110 s, showing a fairly typical spread of contrast, although it is patchy and attenuated in places. The L3–4 and 4–5 transforaminal nerve spill is arrowed in blue.

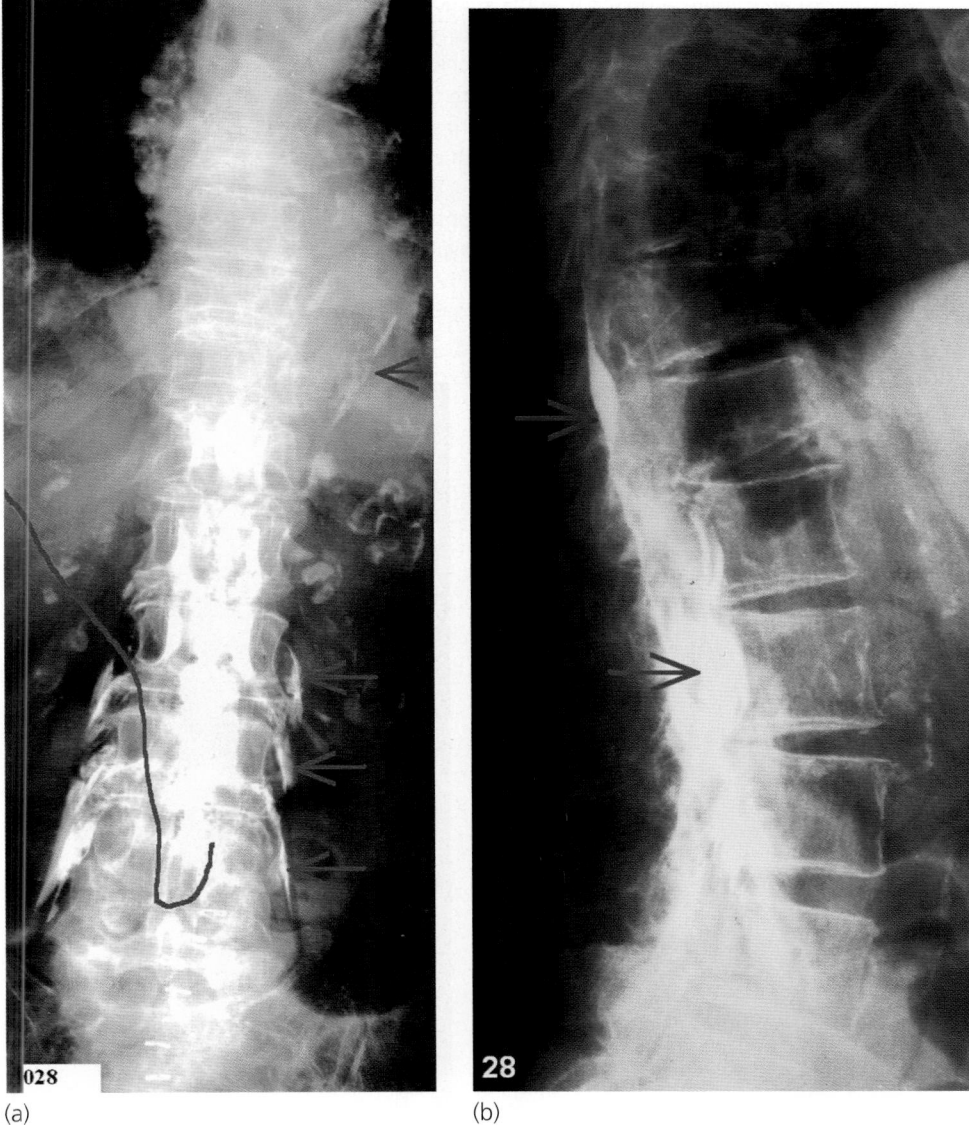

(a) (b)

● **Fig. 3.10** (a) Anteroposterior (AP) epidurogram in an elderly patient with kyphoscoliosis. There are widespread bony degenerative changes, and extensive transforaminal spill of contrast (arrowed on left), the left L1 spill being mostly cephalad (upper arrow). (b) Lateral epidurogram showing a marked kyphosis. There is a high posterior column of contrast and pooling of contrast in some areas (arrowed).

with many pools of contrast appearing, particularly in the posterior column.

Figure 3.11a is an epidurogram following gynaecological surgery on a 77-year-old patient. Satisfactory epidural blockade developed following L2–3 puncture and use of a 19-gauge catheter (Arrow International, Reading, PA, USA) with a flexible tip and a terminal hole. In the AP epidurogram (Fig. 3.11a) there is kyphoscoliosis with widespread degenerative changes in the vertebral bodies. The catheter tip is at L2 in the midline and extensive contrast is seen from T2 to L3, with a patchy spread and

good foraminal spill at several levels. The mass of contrast between T12 and L3 runs across the whole width of the epidural space, but above T12 the column of contrast starts to taper off considerably and there is little foraminal spill. This upper appearance is typical of a posterior distribution of contrast.

The lateral view confirms this (Fig. 3.11b), as a marked posterior column is seen to run from T12 to T2, along a kyphotic curve with an acute angle at T9 (arrowed). Below T12 there is a fairly uniform spread of contrast across the epidural space.

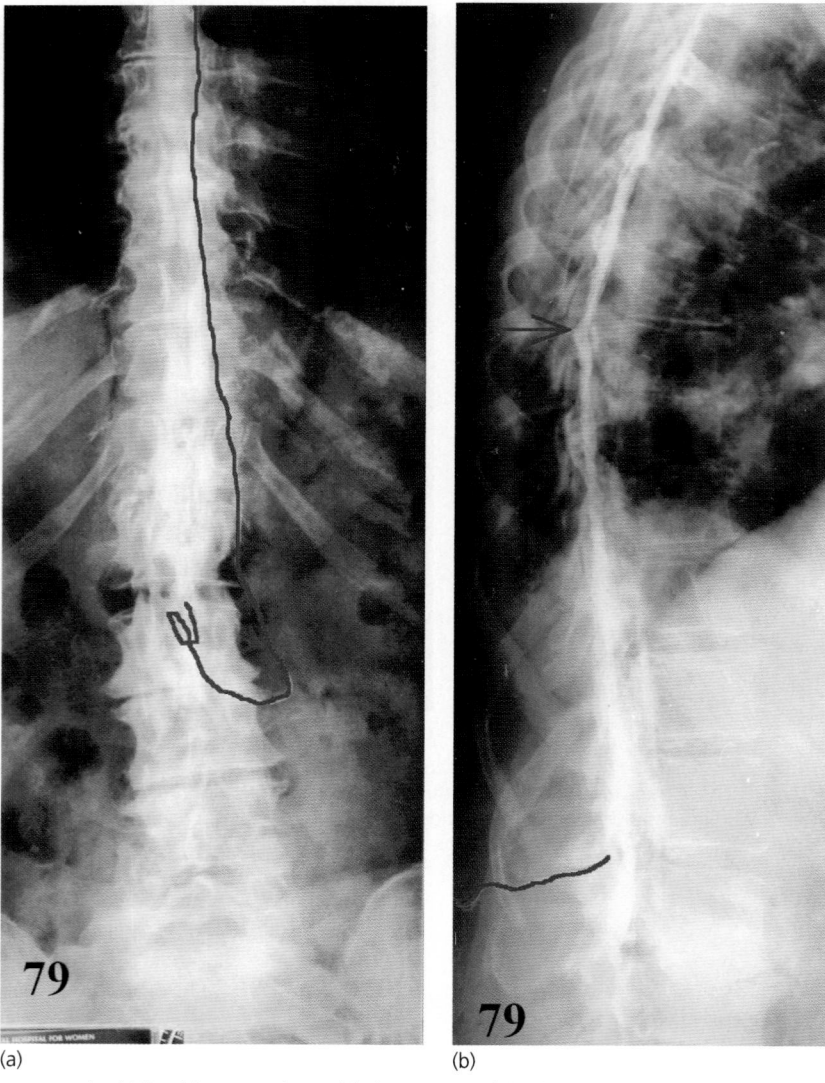

(a)　　　(b)

● **Fig. 3.11** (a) Anteroposterior (AP) epidurogram in an elderly patient with kyphoscoliosis. There are widespread bony degenerative changes. The central aggregation of contrast is narrow and there is little transforaminal spill, suggesting a predominantly posterior distribution of contrast. (b) Lateral epidurogram showing a marked kyphosis, and confirming the extensive and mostly posterior distribution of contrast, with an acute mid-thoracic angulation (arrowed).

3.4 Computed tomography epidurograms

The use of CT scanning allows an accurate assessment to be made as to the precise location of the tip of an epidural catheter following contrast injection,[2] whether it be in the epidural, subdural, or subarachnoid spaces. At present, the intradural space cannot be differentiated. The characteristic axial (horizontal plane) scan appearance of contrast in the epidural space is shown in Fig. 3.12, where subdural contrast is also present. The scan was taken at the level of the L2–3

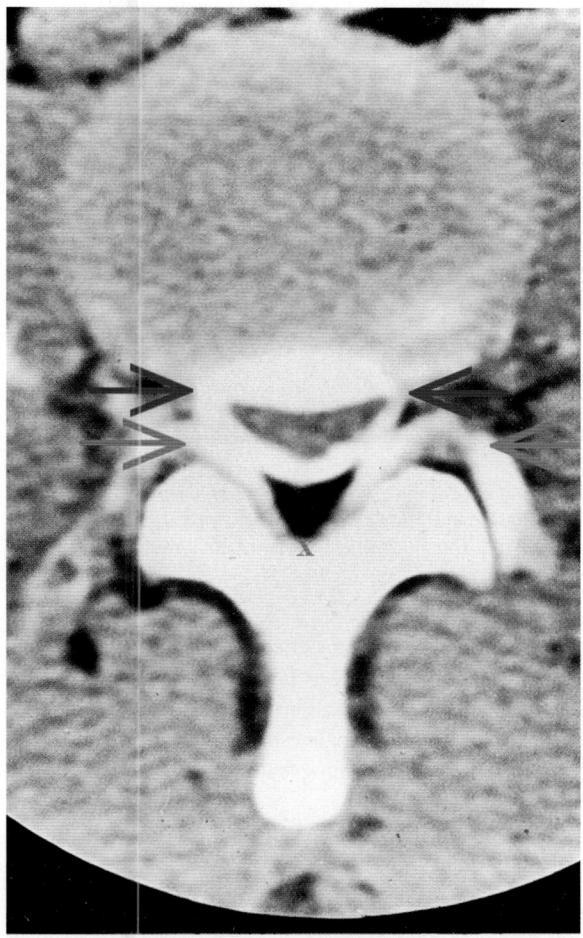

● **Fig. 3.12** Axial computed tomography (CT) scan at L3 showing epidural contrast escaping from the posterior epidural space (X) through both intervertebral foramina (red arrows). Subdural contrast (blue arrows) encloses the nerve roots of the cauda equina.

intervertebral foramina and displays contrast filling the space around the spinal nerves, and spilling into the paravertebral space. At this level the other major feature is the triangular defect, which appears black, occupying almost the whole of the posterior epidural space. This fibro-fatty structure may be associated with obstructive septal barriers. The static axial or longitudinal scans only provide a 'snapshot' of the true picture, and until real-time CT scanning becomes more widely available, X-ray fluoroscopy will remain the only simple means of studying the dynamics of contrast flowing through epidural catheters.

3.5 Magnetic resonance imaging epidurograms

As previously mentioned, magnetic resonance imaging (MRI) scans may be used without contrast to display the contents of the epidural space. As with CT, at present only a static image is presented, but following injection of contrast, catheter tip location can usually be determined. This may be particularly helpful in cases of suspected multicompartment block.

The T1-weighted axial scan using a Signa scanner (General Electric) operating at 1.5 Tesla in a thin healthy supine subject (Fig. 3.13a) clearly shows the triangle of fibro-fatty tissue at the back of the epidural space (arrowed), which appears white, as opposed to black on the previous CT scan. Laterally, the borders of the epidural space are very poorly defined. Fat accompanying the emerging L3 nerves through the intervertebral foramina is also seen. The sagittal scan of the same subject (Fig. 3.13b) shows anterior epidural fat at L5 and the sacrum, but no other evidence of an anterior epidural space, while the posterior epidural space is seen to be incomplete, with white triangles of fat positioned between the vertebral laminae to give a saw-tooth appearance. The possible association between the presence of adipose or fibro-fatty tissue in the posterior epidural space and obstruction to the flow of epidural solutions is discussed in Chapter 7.

3.6 Conclusions

The 'typical' epidurogram is a very variable entity in terms of the vertical extent of contrast spread, as well as the degree of lateral filling of the epidural space and the transforaminal flow, when judged from radiographic plates. Fluoroscopic screening adds an extra dimension, allowing recognition of a characteristic fairly rapid epidural filling pattern, which does not ascend as quickly as subdural spread or as extensively as subarachnoid injection. Multicompartment blocks may be

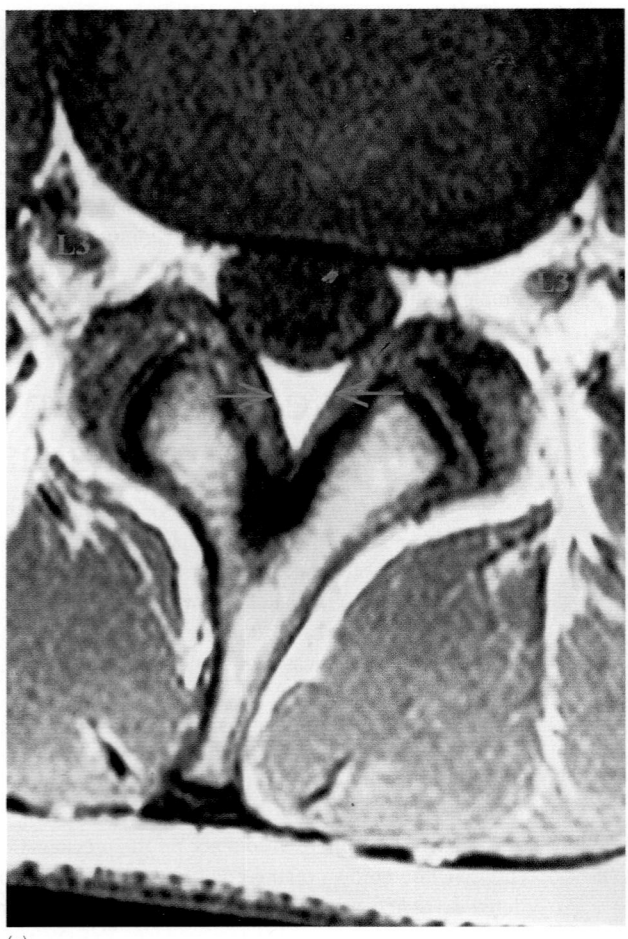

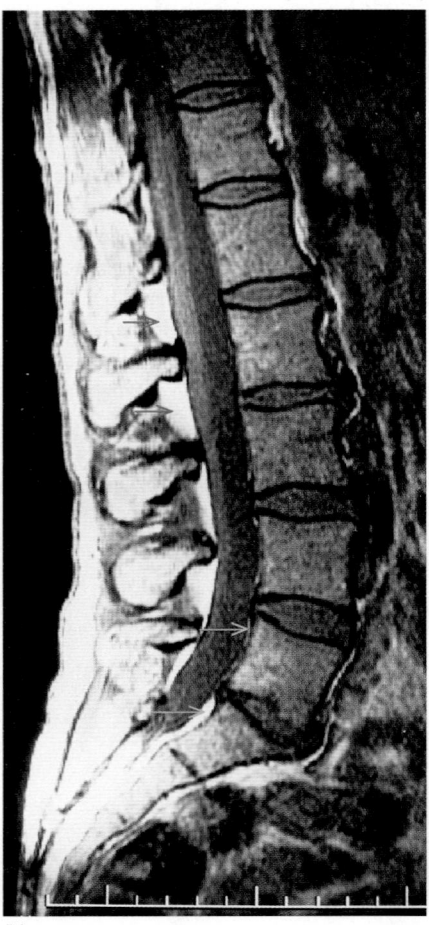

(a)   (b)

● **Fig. 3.13** (a) A typical axial magnetic resonance imaging (MRI) scan at the level of the L3 lamina, without contrast. The posterior epidural space (red arrows) is medial to the ligamentum flavum and vertebral lamina. The L3 nerve roots are indicated. (b) A typical sagittal lumbosacral MRI scan, with the posterior epidural space arrowed in red. The much smaller anterior epidural space is arrowed in blue.

extremely difficult to diagnose, and this is where CT and MRI scans may prove invaluable.

As many investigators have pointed out, attempts to demonstrate a correlation between radiological and clinical spread can produce conflicting results, particularly when the older more viscous ionic contrast media were in use. Now, while the level of neuraxial block, as assessed clinically, is frequently similar to the contrast level seen on radiography, there may be marked differences. However, the two fairly consistent findings would appear to be:

1 The neuraxial block, as assessed clinically, tended to spread further than the contrast indicated, bearing in mind that the volume of local anaesthetic injected was usually larger than the volume of contrast.

2 The development of an effective epidural block at any particular segmental level (apart from the sacral nerves), appeared to correlate well, in most cases, with the presence of at least a small volume of contrast surrounding the corresponding emerging spinal nerve roots.

REFERENCES

1 Magides AD, Sprigg A, Richmond MN (1966) Lumbar epidurography with multi-orifice and single orifice catheters. *Anaesthesia*; 51:757–763.
2 Hogan QH (1999) Epidural catheter tip position and distribution of injectate evaluated by computed tomography. *Anesthesiology*; 90: 964–970.

3 Boezaart AP, Levendig BJ (1989) Epidural air-filled bubbles and unblocked segments. *Canadian Journal of Anaesthesia*; 36:603–604.

4 Dalens B, Bazin J, Haberer J (1987) Epidural bubbles as a cause of incomplete analgesia during epidural anesthesia. *Anesthesia and Analgesia*; 66:679–683.

5 Seeling W, Tomczak R, Merk J, Mrakovcić N (1995) Comparison of conventional and computed tomographic epidurography with contrast medium using thoracic epidural catheters. *Anaesthetist;* 44:24–36.

6 Hogan QH (1991) Lumbar epidural anatomy. A new look by cryomicrotome section. *Anesthesiology*; 75:767–775.

7 Igarashi T, Hirabayashi Y, Shimizu R *et al.* (1997) The lumbar extradural structure changes with increasing age. *British Journal of Anaesthesia*; 78:149–152.

CHAPTER 4
COMPLICATED EPIDURAL BLOCKS

The radiological features of the early major complications of epidural block, whether high epidural,[1] subdural,[2] intradural,[3] subarachnoid,[4] or intravascular injection,[5] have all been described in the anaesthetic literature, either as isolated case reports or review articles. These conditions are of importance as they may cause considerable alarm to patients and staff as well as being occasionally life-threatening. These complications may occur either in isolation, as single-compartment blocks, or less commonly in combination as multicompartment blocks,[6] which typically occur when multi-orifice catheters are in use.

Complicated blocks will be described under the following topics:

1 Intravascular injection
2 High epidural block
3 Accidental subarachnoid (spinal) block
4 Multicompartment block with and without CSF leakage
5 Horner's syndrome
6 Intradural block
7 Subdural block

We have discovered so many examples of intradural and subdural blocks, that a separate chapter (5) has been devoted to them.

4.1 Intravascular injection

Intravascular injection of even a small volume of high-concentration epidural local anaesthetic, as used for caesarean section, is so readily recognized on clinical grounds that further investigation is difficult to justify. However, we have noted two cases where the tip of the epidural catheter was almost certainly partially in the epidural space and partially in an epidural vein, probably over the course of several hours, while a low-dose local anaesthetic infusion was running in labour. In retrospect, both patients reported being unusually 'light-headed' or 'spaced-out', throughout their epidurals in labour, and that their analgesia had been patchy and incomplete. Top-up for emergency caesarean section, with test doses of lidocaine 2%, resulted in the immediate onset of convulsive activity in both patients, confirming at least partial intravascular placement.

The injection of contrast into an epidural vein can be difficult to visualize on screening, with only a very transient faint 'plume' of contrast being seen within 30s of injection, but it is probably worthwhile in the investigation of an unsatisfactory block, although we failed to obtain good quality radiographs in the two patients just described.

4.2 High epidural block

Unusually extensive epidural blocks are quite commonly seen in practice, especially involving obstetric patients and the older local anaesthetic agents. Numbness of the hands and difficulty in breathing are the usual presenting symptoms. Few of these cases are ever investigated.

CASE HISTORY 4.1:
HIGH BLOCK

A 26-year-old (height 152 cm, weight 56 kg) in early labour underwent uneventful epidural block with 18 mL bupivacaine 0.375% administered over a 40-min period. An emergency caesarean section was then required for foetal distress, and a top-up dose of 10 mL lidocaine 2% with adrenaline was given. Ten minutes later, just before delivery, a high block developed. The patient complained of a numb chest (to C4) and numb fingers, with an inability to breathe and a considerable degree of panic, including a feeling of impending death, despite repeated reassurance. The block extended as high as the trigeminal nerves (Fig. 4.1a), with numb cheeks and loss of the corneal reflex bilaterally, before regressing to T4 over a further 20 min. There was no evidence of hypotension (minimum BP 110/60) and neither motor block nor changes in pupil size. In view of the fairly slow onset of the block and the presumed intracranial involvement of the trigeminal nerve, the initial diagnosis was a subdural injection.

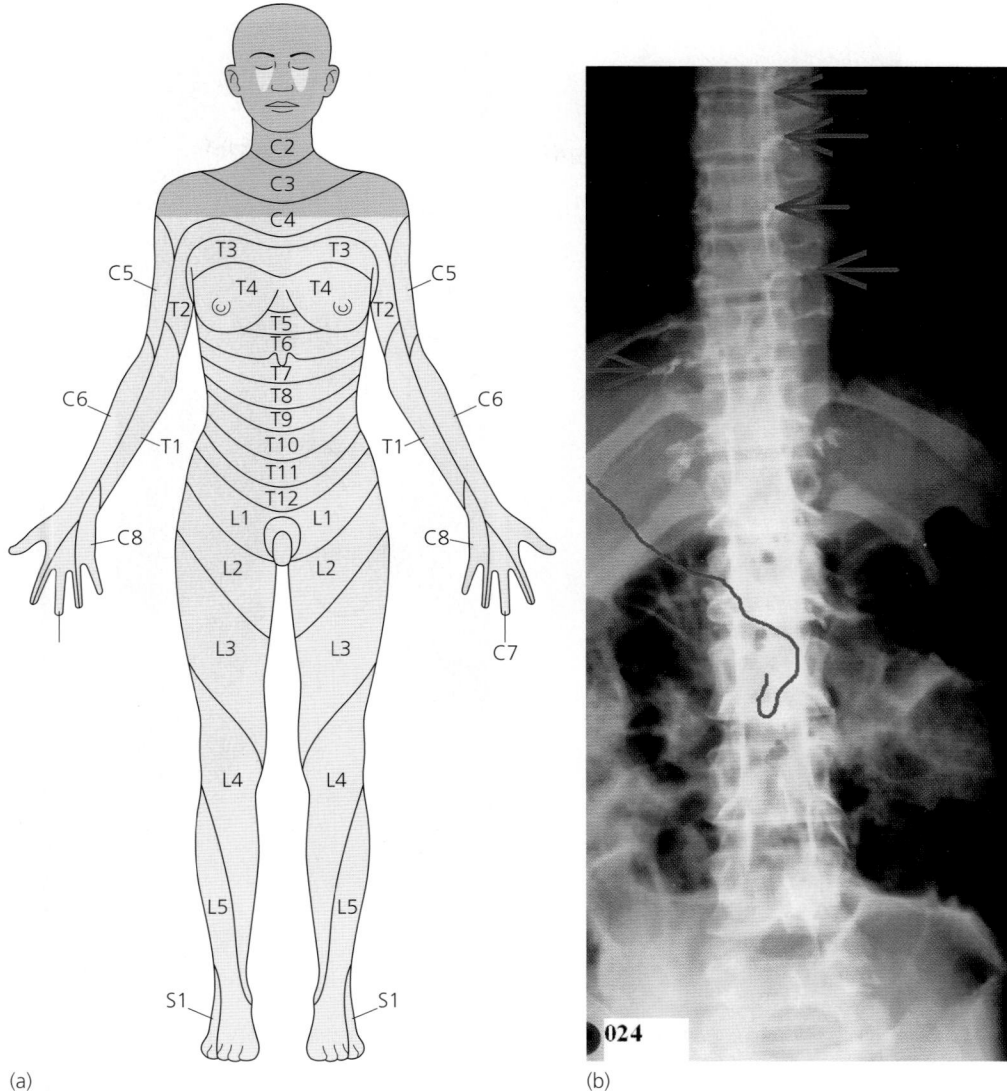

(a)   (b)

● **Fig. 4.1** (a) Dermatomal spread of analgesia to pinprick (lighter-coloured areas) following high epidural block (Case History 4.1), with numb cheeks and loss of corneal reflex from associated bilateral trigeminal nerve block. (b) Anteroposterior (AP) epidurogram in the same patient. Extensive thoracic contrast spread is evident (red arrows), up to T5, with marked transforaminal spill on the left.

Epidurogram findings: **high epidural contrast spread**

On screening, the contrast was seen to be in the epidural space, with excessively high spread, initially in two lateral channels. The anteroposterior (AP) radiograph (Fig. 4.1b) shows the extended 'Christmas-tree' appearance, up to T4 on the left and T7 on the right with transforaminal spill of contrast being unusually abundant in the thoracic spine (red arrows). The catheter tip was located at L2 in the midline. The lateral view (Fig. 4.1c) confirms the extensive vertical spread of the epidural contrast.

This case was almost certainly one of high epidural block, with the trigeminal nerve involvement resulting from blockade of its descending tract at the C2 level.[7] The use of a greater volume of contrast (>10 mL) may have demonstrated higher bilateral thoracic spread.

Follow-up

The same patient presented 4 years later for elective caesarean section under epidural block, which was uneventful following small intermittent doses of local anaesthetic, given over 10 min. The following day, she

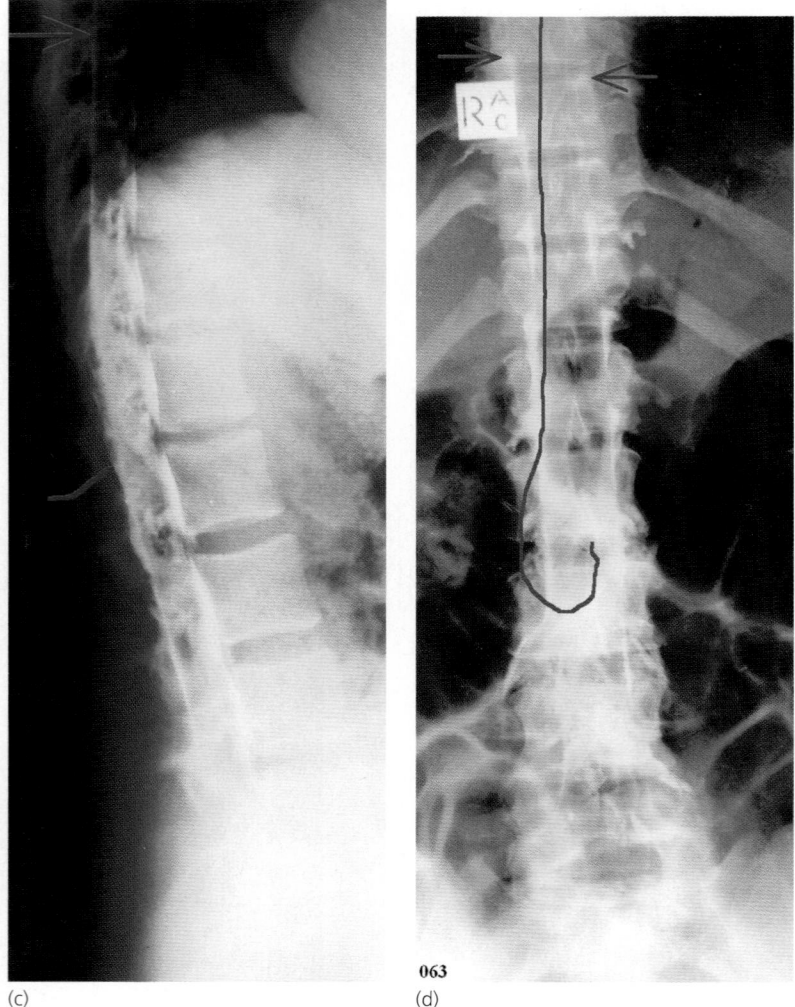

(c)   (d)

Fig. 4.1 (Continued) (c) Lateral epidurogram in the same patient following high epidural block, showing extensive spread of contrast, particularly in the posterior epidural column (red arrow). (d) An AP epidurogram in the same patient 4 years later, showing prominent lateral channels of contrast (arrowed), but not such extensive spread as previously.

consented to epidurography again, in an attempt to explain the cause of the previous high block. The repeat AP screening showed extensive lateral channels of epidural contrast as previously, but only as high as T8, and this time predominantly on the right side, with little central aggregation of contrast (Fig. 4.1d).

The high block and the extensive lateral distribution of contrast on two occasions in this patient, in the absence of an obvious anatomical anomaly, may be attributed to considerable engorgement of the anterior internal vertebral veins at term pregnancy. Such a possibility has been demonstrated by magnetic resonance imaging (MRI) scanning in third-trimester patients in the supine position.[8] In the presence of an obstruction of the inferior

vena cava, these distended veins may tend to encourage the lateral and high spread of epidural solutions. This patient was of short stature and delivered quite large babies, which may have predisposed her to this problem.

4.3 Accidental subarachnoid block

The classical picture of an accidental total spinal (subarachnoid) block, with early and dramatic collapse of the patient accompanied by apnoea and unconsciousness, is usually impossible to mistake for any other situation, especially if cerebrospinal fluid (CSF) can be aspirated through the catheter. However, the current use, in labouring women, of small volumes of dilute solutions of local anaesthetics (usually combined with an opioid) may produce a different and slower sequence of events when injected into the subarachnoid space,[9] and the diagnosis may be difficult, especially if CSF cannot be aspirated, as frequently happens, at least initially.[10] In these situations, or cases of suspected multicompartment or associated intradural block, there is a diagnostic role for epidurography, even when CSF can be freely aspirated. Without investigation, unusual outcomes that may advance our knowledge of the relevant anatomy will be missed, such as an example of contrast spreading from the intradural space to the subarachnoid space in a patient who had presented with a late-onset total spinal block (see Chapter 5).

CASE HISTORY 4.2:
HIGH BLOCK (TO T4)

The patient was a 35-year-old in early labour, who had a 17 g three lateral eye catheter (Portex) introduced to a depth of 5 cm in the epidural space at L4–5. No CSF could be aspirated through the catheter or needle at any time. A test dose of 2 mL lidocaine 2% was injected and within 3 min sensory block was noted at T4 followed by the development of marked motor block in the legs (Bromage grade 3) over the next 5 min. (Throughout this book motor block has been assessed on a modified four-point Bromage scale;[11] grade 0 = no motor block; grade 1 = impaired hip flexion; grade 2 = impaired hip and knee movement; grade 3 = impaired hip, knee and ankle movement.) There was only mild hypotension. A subarachnoid block was suspected and a further 2 mL dose was injected and proved to be an adequate dose for subsequent caesarean section. The block had completely regressed after four hours. Recovery was uneventful, without any headache being reported.

Radiographic findings: subarachnoid contrast
A 2 mL contrast injection was performed 3 h postoperatively, after negative aspiration for CSF. The contrast appeared to be confined to the subarachnoid space, with rapid rostral flow on screening from the midline catheter tip at L4–5 to T4. The AP radiograph (Fig. 4.2a) reveals a very faint narrow and extensive column of contrast, which is featureless apart from some parallel 'linear streaking' representing the emerging nerve roots. Above T12 the contrast image is a little denser and fairly homogeneous, but below this the image becomes very faint as it nears the catheter tip. The total absence of foraminal spill is obvious. Following rotation of the

patient into the left lateral position, contrast is seen to occupy T8–L4 (Fig. 4.2b), again with marked linear streaking.

A further 4 mL of contrast was now injected and both the AP (Fig. 4.2c) and lateral radiographs were repeated (Fig. 4.2d). These revealed consolidation and further vertical spread of the mass of contrast from T6 to L4. Completion of the contrast injection was accompanied by brief discomfort in the L2 dermatome, bilaterally.

CASE HISTORY 4.3:
TOTAL SPINAL BLOCK

A 31-year-old parturient undergoing her fourth caesarean section, and with a history of three difficult and unsatisfactory epidural blocks in her previous pregnancies, developed a suspected total spinal block 7 min after receiving 20 mL ropivacaine 0.875% in four incremental doses over 2 min, through an epidural catheter (Portex 17 g with 3-lateral eyes) at L1–2, following negative aspiration. She collapsed, with moderate hypotension, and became apnoeic. Ventilation was required for 3 h, and the block had totally regressed after 11.5 h. At this time CSF could be freely aspirated. She developed a postdural puncture headache, which was successfully treated with an epidural blood patch.

Radiographic findings: subarachnoid contrast
On the first postoperative day, a dose of 6 mL of contrast was injected and on screening was seen to rapidly spread in the subarachnoid space from T2 to L2. The radiographs (Fig. 4.3) are presented here as negative images for clarity. The AP view (Fig. 4.3a) shows the caudal extension of the contrast (arrowed), which encircled the conus medullaris at L2. This was quite unusual, as this volume of contrast more commonly fills the thecal sac down to S2, as in Fig. 4.6 a,b (p.34). The lateral view (Fig. 4.3b) reveals the characteristic linear streaking of subarachnoid contrast, which had spread to L5 with turning the patient onto her left side.

With this patient's history of poor-quality epidural blocks over several years, and then accidental subarachnoid puncture following a very cautious epidural needle and catheter insertion on this occasion, the possibility arises of scar tissue altering the anatomy of the epidural space and the dura–arachnoid. This would be difficult to visualize radiographically with current techniques, although high-resolution ultrasound (optical coherence tomography) may offer a solution in the future (N. Hoftman, University of California Los Angeles Medical Center, CA, USA, personal communication).[12]

● **Fig. 4.2** (a) Anteroposterior (AP) radiograph following 2 mL of subarachnoid contrast, with a faint appearance of linear streaking from T8 to L1 (arrowed). Note the caudally pointing catheter tip. (b) Lateral radiograph after 2 mL of subarachnoid contrast, with characteristic linear streaking between T8 and L4 (arrowed).

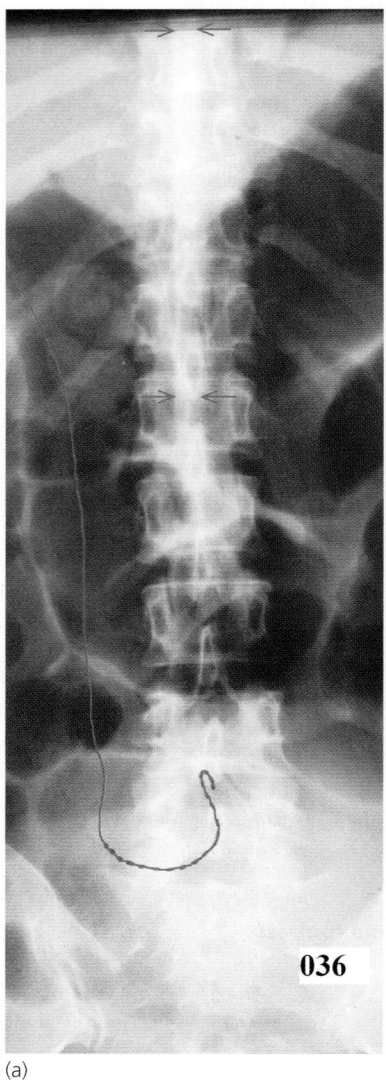

(a)

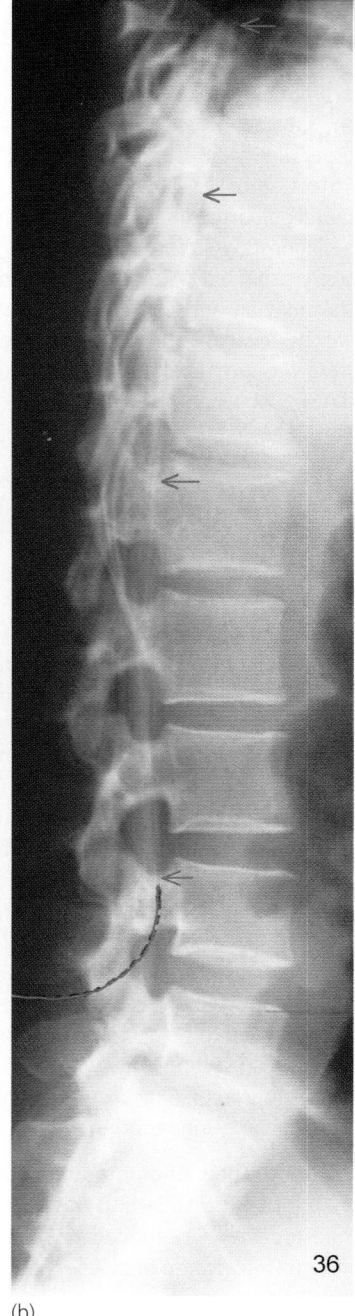

(b)

4.4 Multicompartment block and CSF leakage

So far we have only considered complicated blocks occurring in isolation, apart from the two cases of intravascular/ epidural injection, but less frequently they arise in combination as a multicompartment block.[6] Whereas a combined spinal epidural (CSE) anaesthetic is a planned and usually well-controlled multicompartment block, the unexpected spread of an epidural solution into the subarachnoid, subdural or intradural spaces may produce

● **Fig. 4.2** (Continued) (c) An AP radiograph following 6 mL of contrast, (same patient) with a mass of subarachnoid contrast now extending from T7 to L2 (arrowed). The faint appearance of linear streaking at L2 gradually thickens to a dense mass in the lower thoracic spine. (d) Lateral radiograph following 6 mL of contrast, (same patient) with a mass of subarachnoid contrast extending from T6 to L4 (arrowed). The linear streaking at L4 gradually thickens above, to a denser mass in the lower thoracic spine.

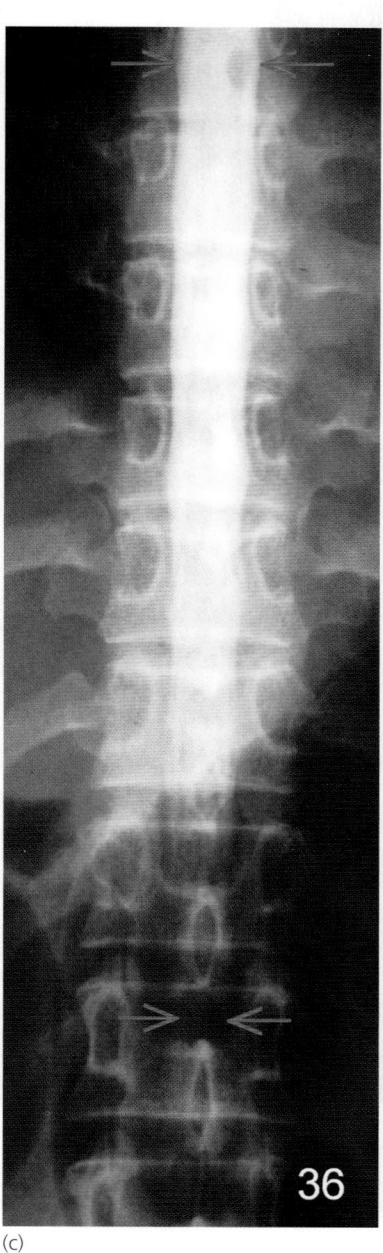

(c)

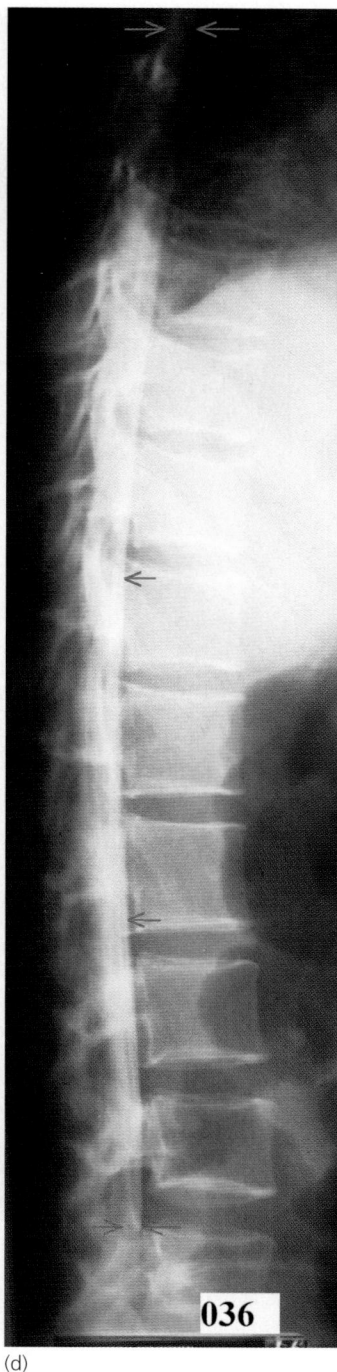

(d)

major complications. The conduit allowing epidural solutions to flow into two or more compartments is, in most cases, a perforation of the dura and sometimes the arachnoid as well.

It is uncertain whether it is more likely for an epidural catheter to be incorrectly inserted with its orifices positioned in two (or very rarely three) of the adjacent compartments (a primary multicompartment block),[6] or for the catheter to migrate into an adjacent space at a later time (a secondary multicompartment block).[13] As the eyes are spaced approximately 4 mm apart in most types

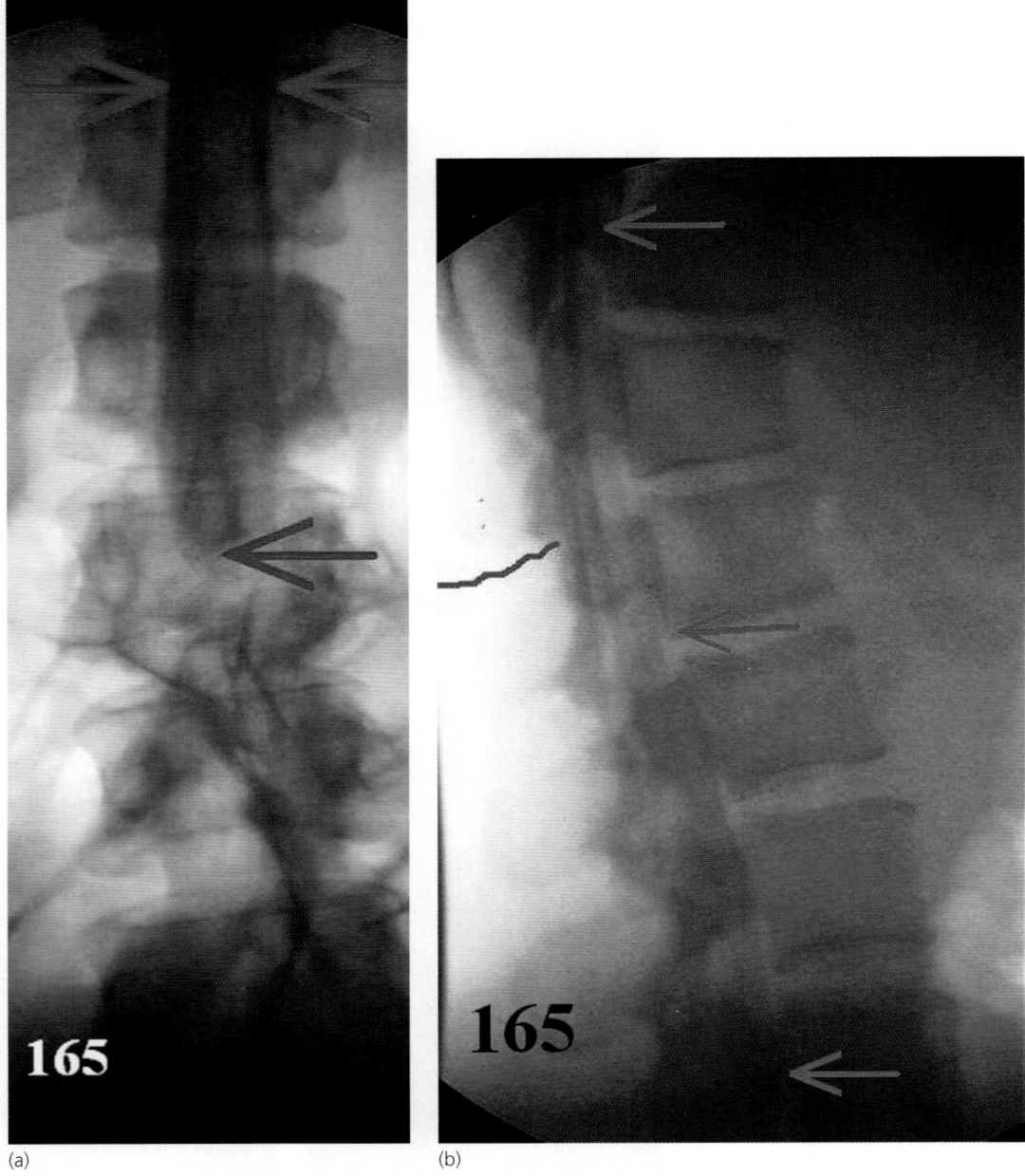

● **Fig. 4.3** (a) Anteroposterior (AP) radiograph (negative image) showing the lower end of an extensive column of subarachnoid contrast, at the level of the conus medullaris, L2, extending up to T12 (arrowed). (b) Lateral radiograph (negative image) showing an extensive column of subarachnoid contrast with faint linear streaking from T12 to L5 (arrowed), following turning of the patient.

of three-hole catheters and the mean thickness of the dura is approximately 0.5 mm, there is always a possibility of multicompartment positioning (Fig. 4.4). However, multicompartment blocks are also possible via epidural needles and single hole or terminal eye catheters (Fig. 4.5).

One of our epidural/intravascular injections was through a terminal eye catheter.

Epidural blocks that also involve the intradural or subdural spaces appear to be the most common types of multicompartment injections and 13 cases are discussed in

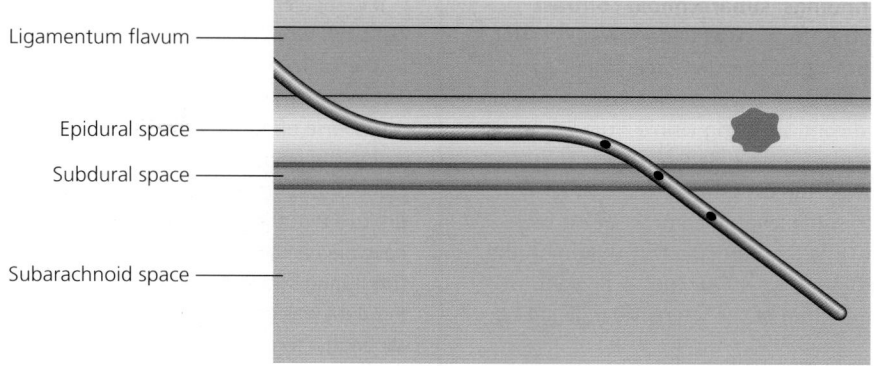

Fig. 4.4 Diagram illustrating the possible positioning of the openings of a typical lateral eye catheter.

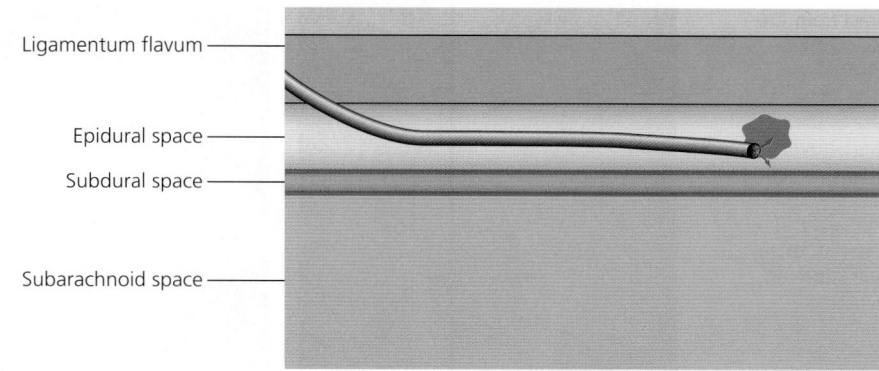

Fig. 4.5 Diagram illustrating the possible multicompartment positioning of the opening of a terminal eye catheter.

Chapter 5. Two cases of combined epidural/subarachnoid block are described here: the first (Case History 4.4) resulted in a high spinal block and the second (Case History 4.5) resulted in a total spinal block.

CASE HISTORY 4.4:
HIGH SPINAL BLOCK (TO T2)

This case appears to be one of those unusual instances where the epidural catheter has entered the subarachnoid space, after an apparently uneventful epidural needle insertion.

A 37-year-old primiparous patient underwent straightforward Tuohy needle insertion at L3–4 prior to elective caesarean section. An initial dose of 15 mL lidocaine 2% with adrenaline administered through the needle produced no ill-effects. Insertion of the epidural catheter (three lateral eyes, 17 g Portex) was difficult,

despite the use of an insertion guide, with passage of the catheter becoming repeatedly obstructed. After several attempts, the resistance was suddenly overcome, with a palpable 'click', and the catheter inserted satisfactorily to a depth of 9 cm. Following fixation of the catheter, aspiration for CSF was negative, and 5 mL of the same local anaesthetic solution was injected 5 min after the initial dose.

After a further 5 min a high block to T2 developed, with dense motor block in the legs and moderate hypotension, which was rapidly corrected with vasopressors. The patient complained of being 'unable to breathe' for approximately 15 min, but this responded to explanation and reassurance. Prior to surgery, blood-stained fluid could be aspirated through the epidural catheter. Caesarean section progressed uneventfully, with the block dissipating after 6 h, when the catheter aspirate was clear fluid. There was no headache reported.

33

Radiographic findings: subarachnoid contrast

Injection of contrast (6 mL) was undertaken 7 h after the block but, unfortunately, the screening images were of poor quality, with only a faint narrow column of subarachnoid contrast being visible from T1 to S2 (Fig. 4.6a), and a dense collection at S2. The AP radiograph showed the catheter tip to be at L3–4 in the midline with subarachnoid contrast being seen to extend from T8 to S2, particularly highlighting the base of the dural sac (Fig. 4.6a). The sacral contrast is also the main feature of the lateral view (Fig. 4.6b, lower arrow).

It is apparent that the epidural catheter penetrated the dura, but whether the dura was intact or already damaged by the Tuohy needle insertion is impossible to determine. The initial dose of lidocaine through the needle produced no adverse effects after 5 min, so was probably retained within the epidural space, suggesting that the epidural catheter itself must have traversed the dura. It appears unlikely that the type of slightly rigid catheter in use could have pierced an intact dura, despite some previous reports suggesting such a possibility,[14] and it is more likely that the dura was damaged by the tip of the Tuohy needle, allowing a forcibly introduced catheter to pass through.[15]

● **Fig. 4.6** (a) Anteroposterior (AP) radiograph showing subarachnoid contrast from T10 to S2 (arrowed). The contrast below L1 is streaky and barely visible, apart from the dense collection at the base of the dural sac at S2 (lower arrow). (b) Lateral radiograph demonstrating dense subarachnoid contrast at the base of the dural sac at S2 (lower arrow). Above this, there is only the faint linear streaking of contrast (upper arrows).

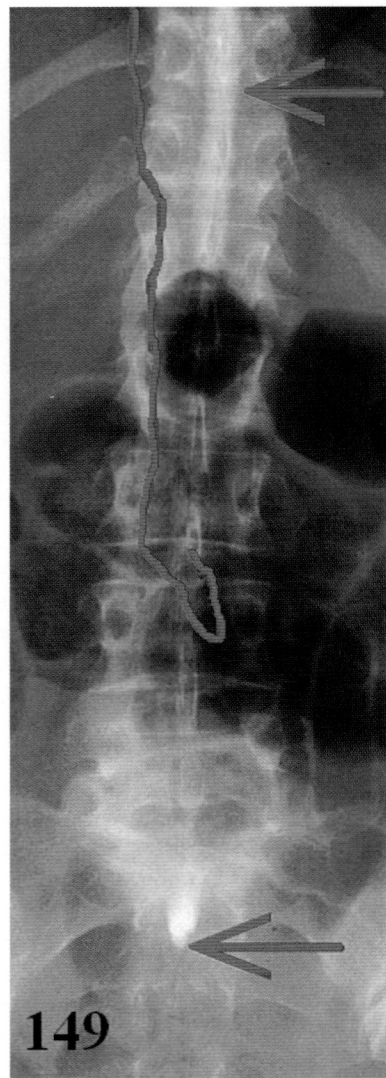

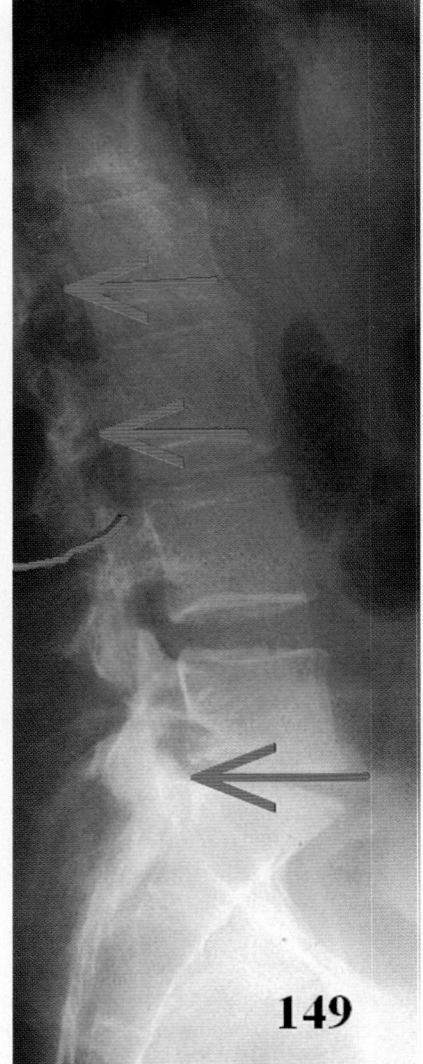

(a)

(b)

CASE HISTORY 4.5:
PATIENT COLLAPSE – TOTAL SPINAL BLOCK

A 49-year-old patient undergoing vaginal repair surgery under regional block, with minimal sedation, had a three lateral eye catheter (17 g, Portex) inserted at L2–3, with 4 cm in the epidural space, and a dose of 15 mL bupivacaine 0.5% was injected. After 15 min, the block was at T8 to pinprick and surgery commenced. Following a further 20 min, with the operation proceeding smoothly, the patient collapsed into unconsciousness with hypotension (systolic blood pressure of 60 mmHg), bradycardia (pulse 45 b.p.m.) and respiratory uncoordination followed by apnoea. The pupils were maximally dilated. Following resuscitation and endotracheal intubation, the patient's lungs were ventilated for the next 2 h, by which time all symptoms had subsided. No CSF could be aspirated.

Epidurogram findings: subarachnoid and epidural contrast

Fluoroscopic screening the following day revealed the presence of marked bony degenerative changes, which were rather advanced for a patient of this age, together with kyphoscoliosis (Fig. 4.7). Following the injection of 4 mL contrast, a dense swelling mass of epidural contrast appeared between T12 and L2. A further 6 mL of contrast appeared to flow into the subarachnoid space as high as T6, followed by further epidural spread from T8–L4, somewhat obscuring the subarachnoid contrast. The AP radiograph (Fig. 4.7) of the lower back showed a typical epidural contrast appearance from T12–L4, with a dense central column of subarachnoid contrast.

Although the history suggested a subdural block, this does appear to be a case of delayed onset of a total spinal block associated with subarachnoid injection through a catheter at least partially within the epidural space. Whether this was a primary or secondary multicompartment block is open to speculation. It is well known that the amount of pressure applied to the plunger of the syringe during administration of local anaesthetic through a multi-hole epidural catheter can determine which orifice receives the preferential flow.[16]

4.4.1 CSF leakage

Whenever there is a hole in the dura there is the possibility of transfer of fluids via this pathway in or out of the subarachnoid space.[17] Two examples of CSF leakage into the epidural space are described in Case History 4.6.

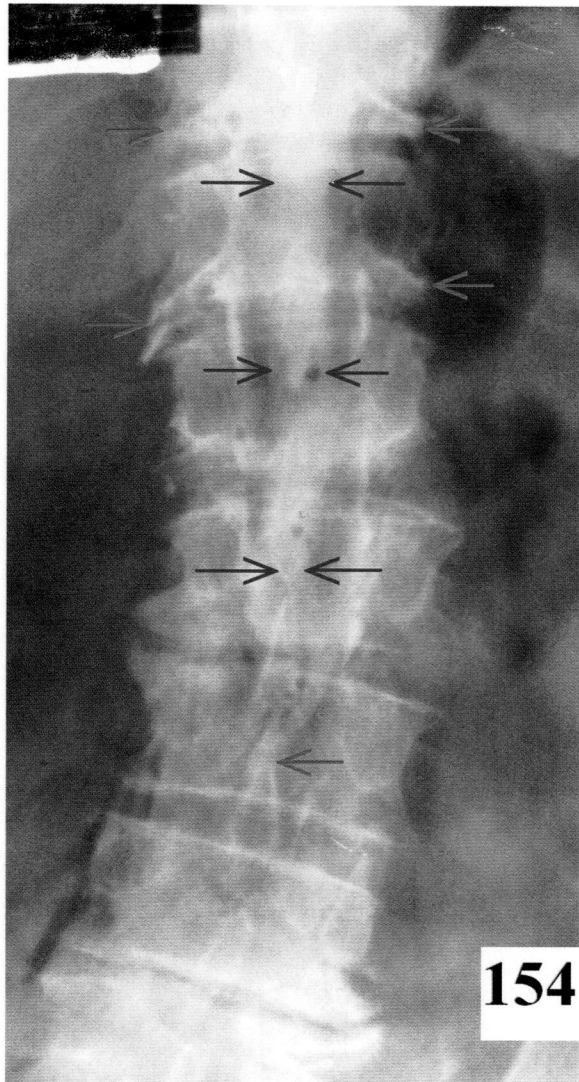

154

● **Fig. 4.7** Anteroposterior (AP) view of a degenerative lower thoracolumbar spine, with epidural contrast from T12 to L4 (lower red arrow) and foraminal spill (upper red arrows). The central subarachnoid mass of contrast (blue arrows) is obscured by epidural contrast at higher vertebral levels.

CASE HISTORY 4.6:
SATISFACTORY CSE AFTER DURAL PUNCTURE

A patient in labour was scheduled for caesarean section and during attempted L2–3 epidural block suffered an accidental dural puncture with a 16-gauge Tuohy needle. A combined spinal epidural (CSE) technique was then performed at L3–4 and surgery was completed successfully after a 2.2 mL dose of heavy bupivacaine 0.5% in glucose 8% was injected into the subarachnoid space, supplemented by epidural 12 mL lidocaine 2% with adrenaline. No CSF could be aspirated through the three lateral eye epidural catheter (Portex) at any time.

Epidurography was undertaken 12 h later, no postoperative epidural analgesia having been administered.

Epidurogram findings: CSF leakage

In the AP view (Fig. 4.8a) the epidural contrast extends from T5 to L4 without foraminal spill, and tapers off

● **Fig. 4.8** (a) Anteroposterior (AP) epidurogram following two dural punctures. The extensive body of epidural contrast is narrowed and contains multiple filling defects (arrowed), almost certainly caused by the accumulation of cerebrospinal fluid (CSF). (b) Lateral epidurogram showing mostly posterior epidural contrast, with a large filling defect anteriorly (upper arrows), presumably due to accumulation of CSF, with an abrupt anterior column cut-off at the top of L4 (lower arrow).

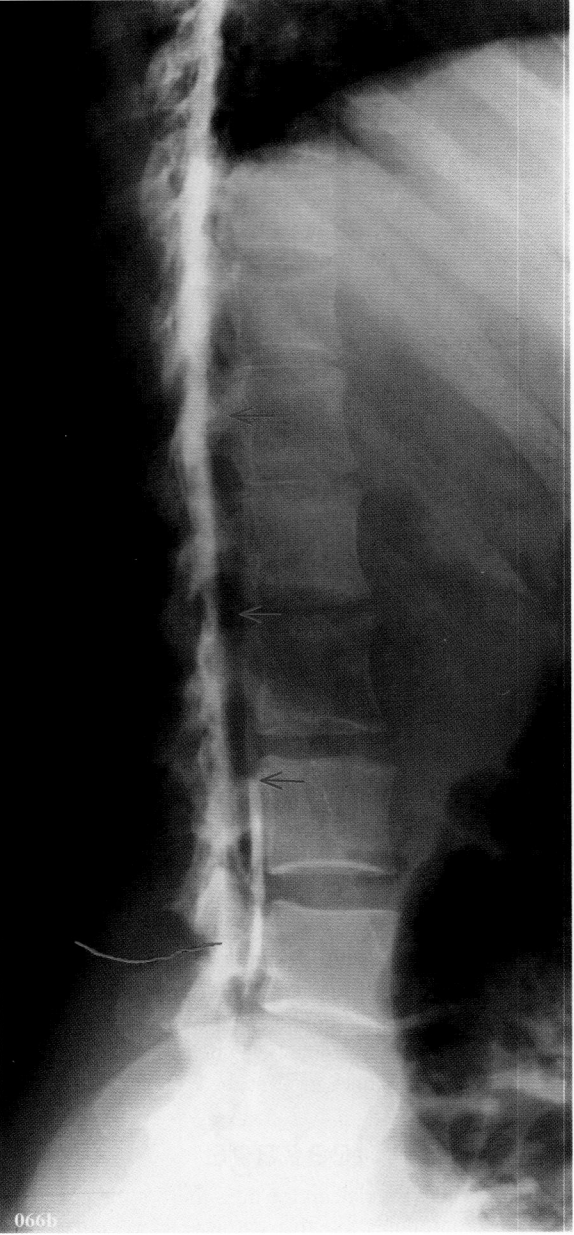

(a) (b)

above and below (indicative of a predominantly posterior distribution). The body of contrast is fragmented by several large filling defects (CSF), most marked at T12, L1 and L2 (Fig. 4.8a, arrowed). The outline of the contrast mass is irregular, blurred and flocculent, as usually seen after recent injection of a local anaesthetic solution. In the lateral view (Fig. 4.8b), the anterior column of contrast is seen to be cut off abruptly above L3 (lower arrow), with an apparently empty anterior space (arrowed). There was no evidence of a lateral septum to cause this maldistribution of contrast. It is presumed that a large volume of CSF had leaked into the epidural space through one or both of the dural puncture sites, as has been reported previously,[16] displacing the epidural contrast posteriorly. It would have been interesting to observe whether postoperative epidural analgesia was successful in this situation, but the catheter was removed immediately after the investigation.

A second example of CSF leakage was well demonstrated by a computed tomography (CT) scan at L3–4 on a patient following a single accidental puncture with a 16 gauge Tuohy needle. Figure 4.9 shows two 'bubbles of fluid' (arrowed). These presumably represent leaked CSF, which appears to occupy a relatively large area of the epidural space. From these and other results,[17,18] it would appear wise to inject epidural solutions with extra caution whenever there is a known accidental perforation of the dura and to closely monitor the progress of the block, as CSF in the epidural space may impede the spread of local anaesthetics.

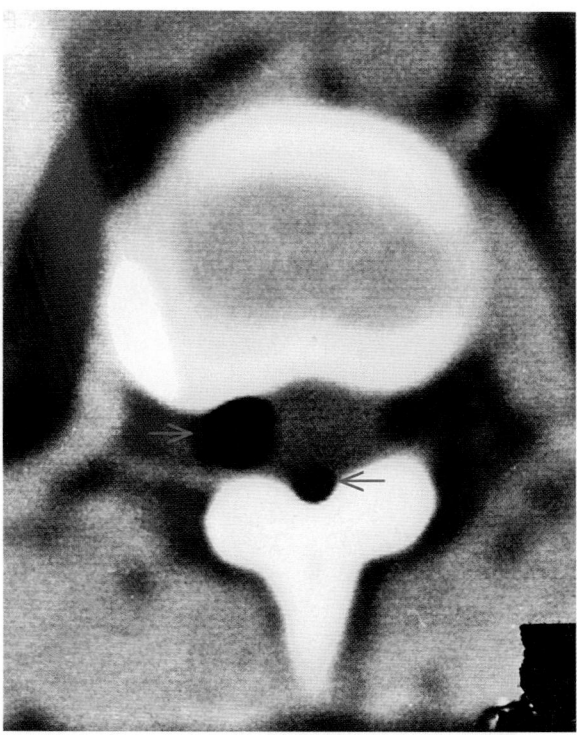

● **Fig. 4.9** Axial computed tomography (CT) scan at L3 with two areas of fluid collection (presumably cerebrospinal fluid) in the epidural space (arrowed) following two dural punctures.

4.5 Horner's syndrome

Horner's syndrome is not uncommonly observed in obstetric patients following lumbar epidural blocks, in two distinct situations. More often it appears as an isolated unexplained finding in the course of a routine block, and less frequently as one component of an excessively high block, particularly in association with a high subdural block,[2] although fixed dilated pupils have also been reported. In our series of 178 epidurogram studies, which specifically investigated high and unusual blocks, seven (4%) of the patients showed unilateral Horner's syndrome, of whom four had clinically high blocks – that is, a sensory level (to blunt pinprick) above T2 – after standard doses of local anaesthetic, with a corresponding high spread of contrast. Of the three patients with Horner's syndrome

following satisfactory blocks, their highest sensory levels recorded were T6, T8 and T10, respectively. It should be noted that the last patient also had spina bifida occulta at S1 and S2.

The full clinical picture of Horner's syndrome, which may rarely be bilateral, consists of ptosis, miosis, enophthalmos and anhidrosis (Fig. 4.10), but not all these components may be present. It is reported as being present in 1–4% of epidural block patients,[19] but is frequently overlooked by medical and nursing staff. Pain in the affected eye,[20] a 'red eye' from dilated conjunctival vessels (Fig. 4.11), or a blocked nose may be the presenting complaint. The symptoms and signs tend to abate within a period of 40 min to 2 h, but may occasionally recur with routine top-up doses, or if a high level of block returns. A recent publication discussed previous recommendations that a block should be abandoned after a Horner's syndrome develops,[21] and concluded that the block should be allowed to proceed, but with caution.

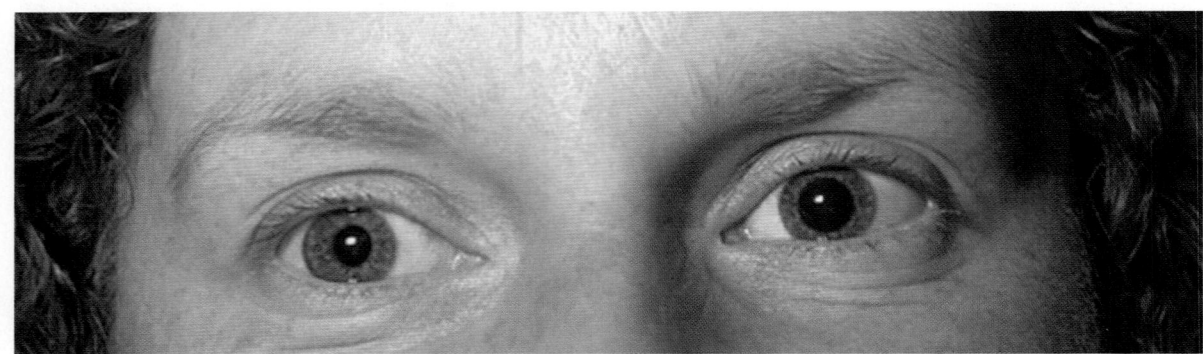

● **Fig. 4.10** Photograph of right Horner's syndrome in a labouring patient. Note the small pupil and slight ptosis.

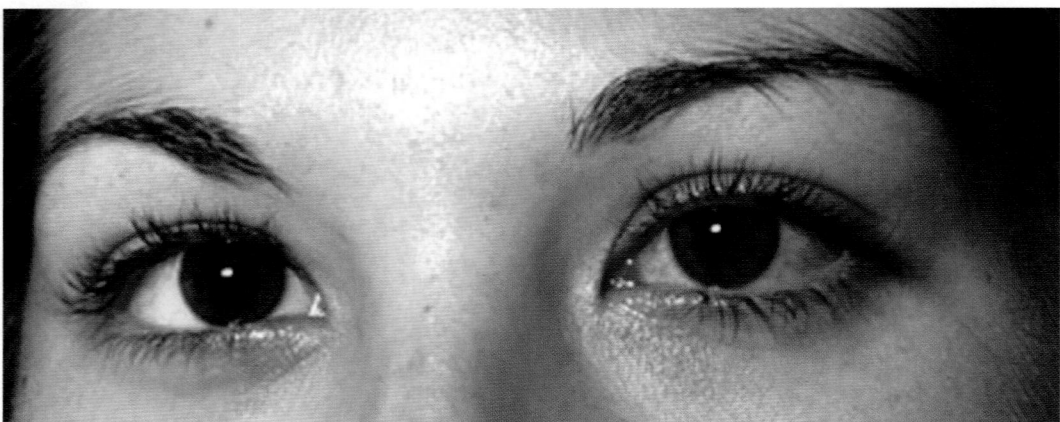

● **Fig. 4.11** Photograph of left Horner's syndrome in a labouring patient, with marked conjunctival injection, miosis and mild ptosis.

The mechanism underlying Horner's syndrome is interruption to the sympathetic nerve supply to the pupil, levator palpebrae muscles, conjunctiva and face. Preganglionic sympathetic fibres emerge predominantly from the upper three thoracic spinal segments, but may also involve the T4 and T5 segments.[22] The fibres then ascend and synapse in the cervical ganglia before reaching the head and neck. The sympathetic fibres are of smaller diameter and are blocked at lower concentrations of local anaesthetic than motor or sensory nerves. This may account for those cases of the syndrome where the upper level of sensory block was well below the T2 level. Figure 4.12 is the epidurogram of a parturient who developed Horner's syndrome during a caesarean section, with a sensory block level never above T6. It shows a normal pattern of contrast spread (10 mL) that did not extend much above T10. More research is required into the exact cause of Horner's syndrome in association with epidural block.

4.6 Conclusions

In summary, many types of complicated block have been described, and there are probably more variations to be discovered. It must be pointed out that investigation of a complicated block may be of little value to the individual patient concerned, as an anatomical abnormality is an unusual finding and the complication is unlikely to recur with subsequent blocks, with certain noted exceptions, such as intradural and subdural blocks. However, with these types of radiological investigation, our overall knowledge of epidural blocks may be consolidated and improvements in techniques and equipment instigated.

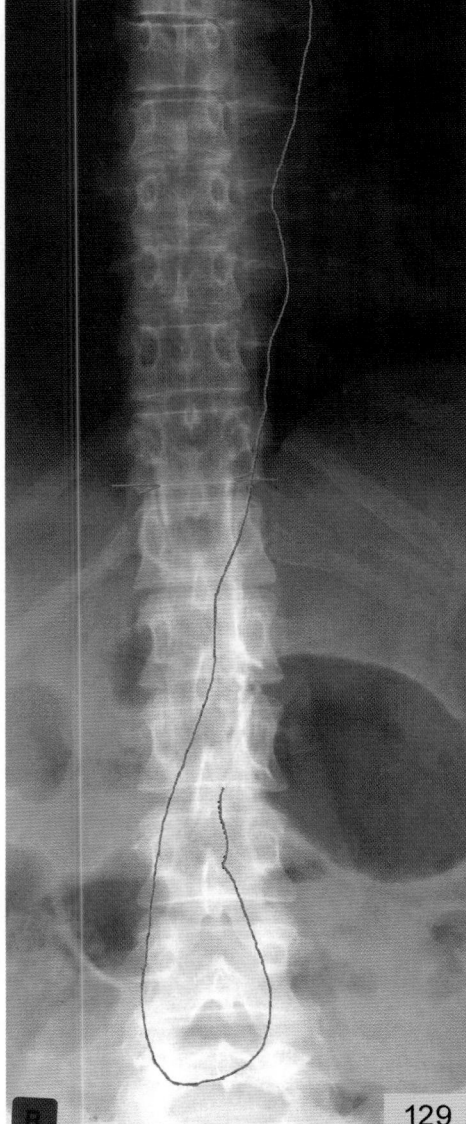

● **Fig. 4.12** Anteroposterior (AP) epidurogram showing a 'normal' spread of contrast, which only ascended to T11/12 (arrowed), in a patient with (right) Horner's syndrome.

REFERENCES

1 Sprung J, Haddox JD, Maitra-D'Cruze AM (1985) Horner's syndrome and trigeminal nerve palsy after lumbar epidural anesthesia. *Anesthesia and Analgesia*; 38:767–771.

2 Hoftman NH, Ferrante FM (2009) Diagnosis of unintentional subdural anesthesia/analgesia: analysing radiographically proven cases to define the clinical entity and to develop a diagnostic algorithm. *Regional Anesthesia and Pain Medicine*; 34:12–16.

3 Collier CB (2010) The intradural space; the fourth place to go astray during epidural block. *International Journal of Obstetric Anesthesia*; 19:133–141.

4 Barnes PK (1990) Delayed subarachnoid migration of an epidural catheter. *Anaesthesia and Intensive Care*; 18:564–566.

5 Crawford JS (1985) Some maternal complications of epidural analgesia for labour. *Anaesthesia*; 40:1219–1225.

6 Beck H, Brassow F, Doehn M et al. (1986) Epidural catheters of the multi-orifice type. Dangers and complications. *Acta Anaesthesiologica Scandinavica*; 30:549–555.

7 Collier CB (1997) Bilateral trigeminal nerve palsy during an extensive lumbar epidural block. *International Journal of Obstetric Anesthesia*; 6:185–189.

8 Hirabayashi JL, Shimizu R, Fukuda H et al. (1996) Soft tissue anatomy within the vertebral canal in pregnant women. *British Journal of Anaesthesia*; 77:153–156.

9 Evans TI (1974) Total spinal anaesthesia. *Anaesthesia and Intensive Care*; 2:158–163.

10 Prince G, McGregor D (1979) Obstetric epidural test doses. A reappraisal. *Anaesthesia*; 41:1240–1250.

11 Phillips GH (1988) Continuous infusion epidural analgesia in labor: effect of adding sufentanil to 0.125% bupivacaine. *Anesthesia and Analgesia*; 67:462–465.

12 Raphael DT, Yang C, Tresser N et al. (2007) Images of spinal nerves and adjacent structures with optical coherence tomography: preliminary animal studies. *Journal of Pain*; 8:767–773.

13 Gregoretti S (1978) Uneventful extradural analgesia after unrecognized dural perforation. *Canadian Anaesthetists Society Journal*; 25:509–511.

14 Hardy PAJ (1986) Can epidural catheters penetrate dura mater? An anatomical study. *Anaesthesia*; 41:1146–1147.

15 Abouleish E, Goldstein M (1986) Migration of an extradural catheter into the subdural space. A case report. *British Journal of Anaesthesia*; 58:1194–1197.

16 Power I, Thorburn J (1988) Differential flow from multihole epidural catheters. *Anaesthesia*; 43:876–878.

17 Collier CB (2000) Complications of Regional Anesthesia. In *International Textbook of Obstetric Anesthesiology*, editors Birnbach D, Gatt SP, Datta S. Churchill Livingstone/Saunders, New York, p. 511.

18 Morgan B (1990) Unexpectedly extensive conduction blocks in obstetric epidural analgesia. *Anaesthesia*; 45:148–152.

19 Clayton RC (1983) The incidence of Horner's syndrome during lumbar extradural for elective Caesarean section and provision of analgesia during labour. *Anaesthesia*; 38:583–585.

20 Abdelatti MO (1993) Horner's syndrome due to epidural anaesthesia presenting with a painful eye. *Anaesthesia*; 48:1019–1020.

21 Hoftman N, Chan K (2009) Two cases of Horner syndrome after administration of an epidural test dose that did not recur with subsequent epidural activation. *Regional Anesthesia and Pain Medicine*; 34:372–374.

22 Zoellner PA, Bode ET (1991) Horner's syndrome after epidural block in early pregnancy. *Regional Anesthesia and Pain Medicine*; 16: 242–244.

CHAPTER 5
THE SUBDURAL AND INTRADURAL SPACES

Considerable uncertainty exists regarding the subject of accidental injection of local anaesthetic into the region commonly referred to as the 'subdural space' during attempted epidural block, particularly in obstetric practice. As most cases are never investigated, the incidence is unknown and an anatomical diagnosis is rarely made. Our radiographic study of 132 parturients with complicated, failed or inadequate epidural blocks revealed 13 instances of contrast injection into the 'subdural region'. In three cases the true subdural space was entered, while in the other 10, it was the adjacent 'intradural' space, an area within the dura previously unrecognized by anaesthetists.

5.1 Accidental subdural injection

In 1990, Reynolds and Speedy described the subdural space as 'the third place to go astray' with an epidural needle or catheter during attempted epidural block (the first two places involving subarachnoid or intravascular invasion).[1] Over the last 30 years there have been numerous reports of accidental subdural injections, some supported by radiographic evidence.[2-8] The clinical features of subdural injection (Table 5.1, left) are the slow onset of a high sensory block, usually 10–35 min after an apparently uneventful epidural

block insertion[7] or even injection of a test dose alone.[8] There may be slow extension of the block over another 15–20 min, sometimes accompanied by dense motor block.[7] As the subdural space may extend into the cranial cavity, and as high as the floor of the third ventricle, extensive spread of local anaesthetic may produce respiratory depression followed by apnoea, and later unconsciousness, with fixed dilated pupils, often accompanied by moderate hypotension.[7] High blocks with an unconscious patient are extremely rare these days because of improved epidural insertion techniques as well as the use in labouring patients of small incremental doses of weak local anaesthetic solutions. Many less extensive cases of subdural block in parturients almost certainly go unrecognized. A sparing of motor and sympathetic block has repeatedly been claimed to be a typical feature of subdural blocks[9] since an isolated case report in 1984;[10] this finding appears to be incorrect on reviewing all the relevant published case histories.[2]

CASE HISTORY 5.1:
TOTAL SUBDURAL BLOCK

This case describes the features of a total subdural block; that is, a block that extends intracranially, with unconsciousness. Considerable clinical details are supplied, as there are very few published cases accompanied by clear radiological evidence, and the features of the block may vary with the particular local anaesthetic in use and its concentration. There also appear to be very few reports of total subdural block with ropivacaine.

A 32-year-old patient (weight 60 kg) was scheduled for repeat elective caesarean section. Insertion of an epidural needle at L3–4 prior to the first operation 15 months previously had resulted in a dural puncture. The needle was withdrawn into the epidural space and a successful block ensued. A mild postdural puncture headache developed on the fifth postoperative day, and gradually worsened, requiring her readmission to hospital and insertion of a blood patch (18 mL) on the seventh day. There were no further problems.

● **Table 5.1** Comparison of the typical features of subdural and intradural block

SUBDURAL BLOCK	INTRADURAL BLOCK
1. Slow onset, over 15–20 min	1. Slow onset, over 20–40 min
2. Gradual progression of block	2. Limited spread, inadequate block initially
3. Exaggerated spread, over further 15–20 min	3. Large total volumes of local anaesthetic required
4. Possible intracranial spread	4. Pain on catheter insertion and top-up may occur
5. Hypotension is moderate (systolic BP usually >80 mmHg)	5. Numbness (dermatomal) may follow intradural pethidine (meperidine)

The time sequence on this occasion was as follows.

Initial block

Following straightforward Tuohy needle introduction at L3–4, the epidural catheter (Arrow International, Reading, PA, USA) met slight transient resistance at the 12 cm mark during insertion, and a 4 cm length was left in the space. A dose of 20 mL ropivacaine 0.875% was given over 2 min.

After 30 min, the block was only as high as T11 to pinprick, with immobile legs (Bromage 3) and cold feet, indicating lack of lumbar sympathetic block. The addition of a further 15 mL of the same local anaesthetic over the next 20 min did not improve the block. (The patient was then offered a general anaesthetic, but declined.)

Second block

- **Elapsed time 00.00:** the L3–4 catheter was removed, having been in place for 60 min. Withdrawal was accompanied by moderate leakage of local anaesthetic back through the skin insertion site, suggesting raised pressure within the epidural space. Another epidural needle was inserted uneventfully at L2–3, following negative aspiration, and 15 mL of the same local anaesthetic given through the needle over 60 s and a catheter inserted to 4 cm
- **+00.20:** within 5 min of injection, the block was at T4 to pinprick and surgery commenced, with no discomfort
- **+00.29:** baby delivered in good condition
- **+00.33:** patient unable to move her arms or hold the baby, and unable to see clearly. Pupils noted to be dilated and fixed, but patient conversing freely! Respiration unimpeded, oxygen saturation (SpO$_2$) = 100% on room air. Block level at C4
- **+00.40:** breathing becoming uncoordinated, with increasing diaphragmatic component
- **+00.45:** SpO$_2$ falling briefly to 60% with gradually decreasing respiratory movements, then apnoea, with unconsciousness. Intermittent positive pressure ventilation applied by face mask, then laryngeal mask airway. SpO$_2$ rapidly restored to 100%
- **+00.55:** surgery completed, patient apnoeic and unconscious but stable. No falls in systolic blood pressure below 100 mmHg were recorded at any time
- **+01.05:** trachea intubated without patient responding, prior to transfer to intensive care unit
- **+01.20:** spontaneous ventilation resumed
- **+01.25:** patient biting on endotracheal tube, which was removed. Patient awake and responding, but still with dilated pupils

- **+02.30:** pupils restored to normal size and reactive, together with return of slight right arm movement
- **+03.30:** full strength returned to arms, right leg moving (Bromage 1)
- **+08.00:** block fully regressed, with complaints of postoperative pain commencing. PCEA (patient controlled epidural anaesthesia) with pethidine 15 mg (3 mL) boluses with 20 minute lockout proved effective
- **+18.00:** epidural contrast injection undertaken with fluoroscopy

The condition was explained to the patient, who was amnesic for the whole operation and made an uneventful recovery.

Epidurogram findings: posterior epidural contrast with anterior subdural leakage

Anteroposterior (AP) fluoroscopy revealed the catheter tip to be in the midline at L3. Initial contrast injection produced a dense irregular mass of contrast at L1–3 (Fig. 5.1a), with irregular edges, and enclosing many air bubbles. As the mass enlarged, contrast (appearing black) flowed around the right L1/2 and L2/3 nerve roots (red arrows), and later extended down to L5 as a faint, patchy collection, again with numerous air bubbles. The AP radiograph (Fig. 5.1a) is suggestive of a restricted posterior epidural distribution of contrast but also shows very faint narrow bilateral columns of subdural contrast (blue arrows), which were not detectable on AP screening. The left subdural column extends from T6 to L1 and the right from T6 to T10, although partly obscured by the epidural catheter.

The lateral view (Fig. 5.1b) demonstrates the epidural catheter entering a restricted posterior mass of contrast extending from L1 to L5, typical of the distribution most commonly seen as a result of adhesions following spinal surgery. In addition, there is a fine, bright anterior column of subdural contrast (blue arrows) which extended as high as T6 on lateral screening.

While this patient may have had a congenital septum, it seems more likely that there was scarring from the previous epidural blood patch, forming a barrier that restricted the flow of local anaesthetic, although it has been demonstrated in animal studies that an epidural blood patch should dissipate within a couple of weeks, with minimal scarring.[11] However, the first dose of epidural local anaesthetic (L3–4) did not spread sufficiently rostrally, presumably because of the septum acting as an obstruction, while allowing a collection of local anaesthetic to accumulate below it. The second epidural needle insertion (L2–3) almost certainly entered the same space and further local anaesthetic injection resulted in a

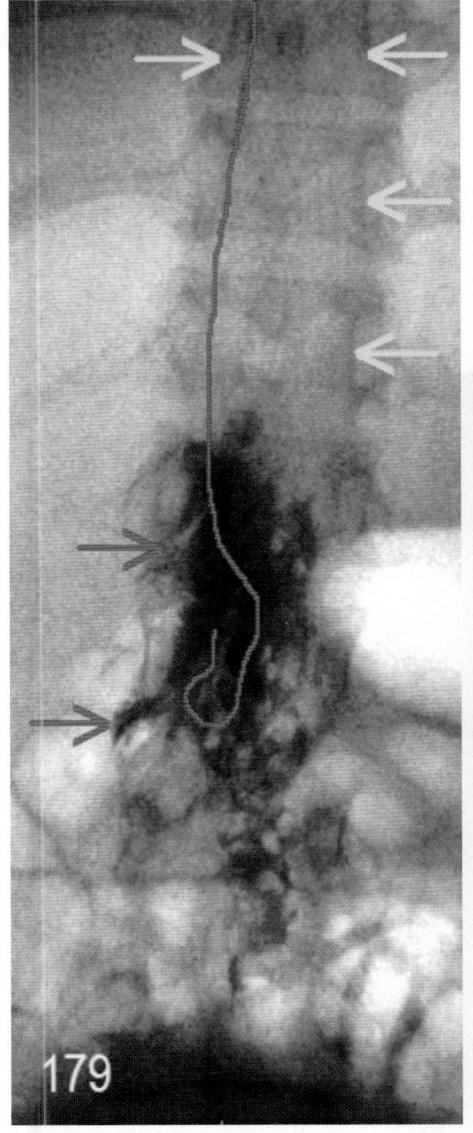

(a)

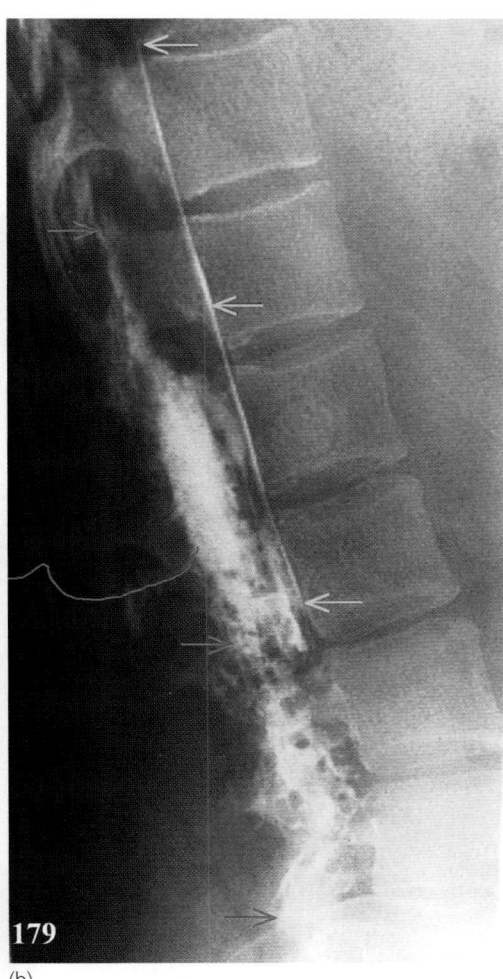

(b)

● **Fig. 5.1** (a) Anteroposterior (AP) epidurogram revealing a dense mass of mostly right-sided epidural contrast (here appears black) at L1-L3, with an irregular edge and containing many air bubbles. Contrast also highlights the right L1–2 and L2–3 nerve roots (red arrows). Very faint columns of subdural contrast are visible from T6 to L1 on the left and T6 to T10 on the right (blue arrows), although the latter is partly obscured by the epidural catheter. (b) Lateral epidurogram showing the posterior epidural collection of contrast between L1 and L3 (red arrows) and a narrow anterior dense column of subdural contrast from T6 to L3.

build-up of pressure that almost certainly caused rupture of the dura, but not the arachnoid. A subdural space was created and an intracranial block resulted.

CASE HISTORY 5.2:
HIGH SUBDURAL BLOCK (TO T2)

Prior to an emergency caesarean section on a 31-year-old primiparous patient, a Tuohy needle was inserted

without difficulty into the epidural space at L2–3, and 4 mL lidocaine 2% with adrenaline injected. A catheter with three lateral eyes (Portex Ltd, Ashford, Kent, UK) was then inserted to a depth of 3 cm in the space and, following negative aspiration, a further 4 mL with 40 μg fentanyl was given. Fifteen minutes later, the upper level of sensory block was at T2, with immobile legs (Bromage 3) and the systolic blood pressure

(BP) had fallen to 70 mmHg. Intravenous ephedrine (total dose = 15 mg) restored the BP and surgery was performed satisfactorily over the course of 1 h, after a total of only 8 mL of 'epidural' local anaesthetic.

The clinical diagnosis, at that stage, was considered to be either a subdural or a subarachnoid block and after some deliberation it was decided to proceed carefully with our standard postoperative continuous epidural infusion (at that time) of 0.1% bupivacaine. A small dose

of 0.5–1.0 mL/h provided excellent analgesia, without any complications. Contrast injection was undertaken next day.

Epidurogram findings: bilateral subdural contrast

On screening, the rapid filling of two narrow, lateral columns of contrast (Fig. 5.2a) was the most striking feature. The flow of contrast was much faster than that seen following epidural injection. In the AP

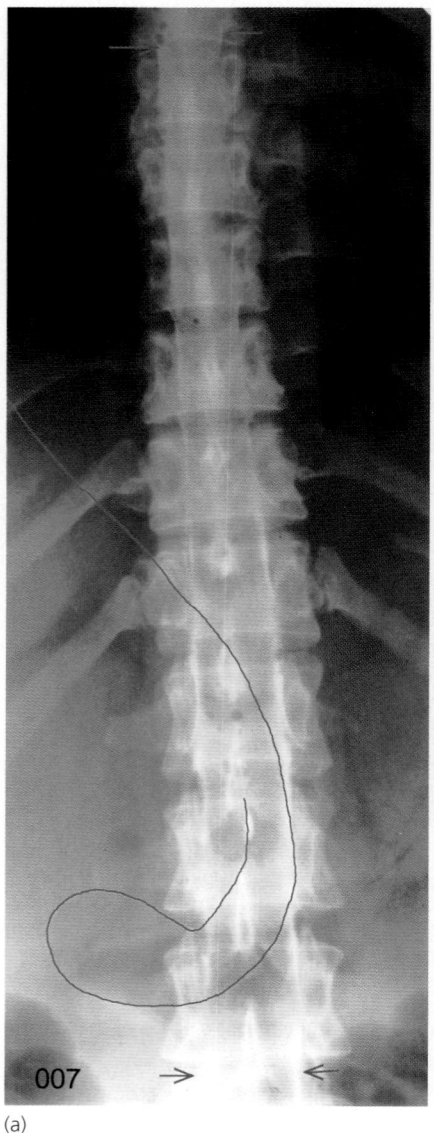
(a)

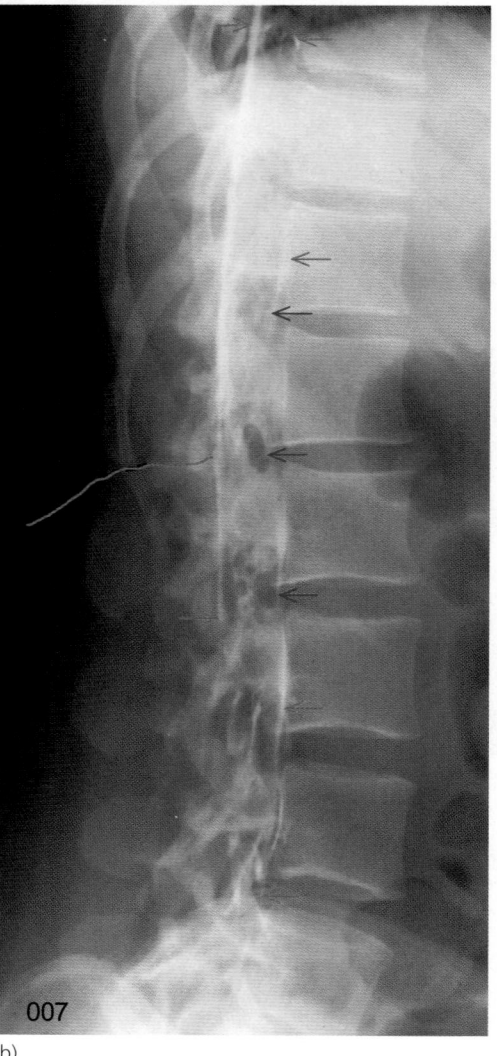
(b)

● **Fig. 5.2** (a) Anteroposterior (AP) epidurogram, following a high block, revealing bilateral subdural columns of contrast from T4 to L4 (arrowed), with a 'rail-road track' appearance. (Reproduced from Collier CB, Gatt SP, Lockley SM. *Br J Anaesth* 1993; 70:462–465 with the kind permission of Oxford Journals and the authors). (b) Lateral epidurogram showing anterior and posterior columns of subdural contrast (red arrows) with a small volume of contrast in between. The intervertebral foramina (blue arrows) are characteristically empty.

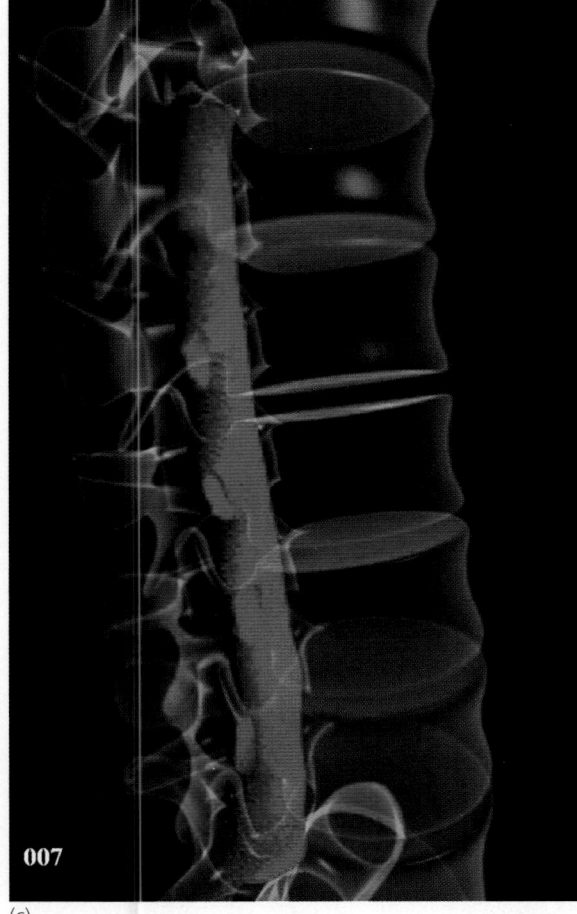

007

(c)

● **Fig. 5.2** (Continued) (c) Three-dimensional modelling of the radiographs from the same patient (3D Studio Max).

radiograph (Fig. 5.2a), the catheter tip is seen to be at L2 in the midline, with the typical picture of subdural contrast flowing from T4 to L4, creating a 'rail-road track' appearance of parallel columns of contrast in the thoraco-lumbar area. This pattern of contrast distribution appears to result from the subdural space tending to spread laterally as it opens up (see later) and accounts for the preferential accumulation of contrast adjacent to the spinal nerve roots.

There is also a sharp lateral cut-off to the flow of contrast, which does not extend beyond the vertebral bodies, and there is no foraminal spill. The faint shadowing in the midline, between the lateral columns, represents the spread of a small volume of subdural contrast around the catheter tip.

In the lateral view (Fig. 5.2b), there are faint anterior and posterior columns of contrast, from T4 to L4 (red arrows), with patchy contrast between. A diagnostic feature is that the intervertebral foramina are virtually empty, as there is no contrast escaping from either the epidural or subdural spaces, and the nerve roots are not highlighted. Three-dimensional modelling based on the radiographs of this patient resulted in the image shown in Fig. 5.2c (see accompanying website for moving images).

In Case History 5.3 the subdural block was predominantly unilateral.

CASE HISTORY 5.3:
HIGH SUBDURAL BLOCK (TO C4)

A lateral eye catheter (Portex) was inserted at the L2–3 interspace in a primiparous labouring patient and a dose of 10 mL bupivacaine 0.25% was injected. After 30 min a high block had developed, with numbness of the arms, and the chest up to the clavicles (C4), together with weakness of the right hand. A few minutes later, the patient reported a tingling sensation in the right side of the face. On examination, there was loss of sensation to pinprick over the trigeminal nerve area, with loss of corneal reflex, but no Horner's syndrome or pupillary changes. Both legs developed moderate motor block (Bromage 2). All symptoms had regressed after a further 45 min, and no further local anaesthetic was injected, as delivery was imminent. Six hours later, contrast injection was undertaken.

Epidurogram findings: right subdural contrast (predominantly)

On screening following 6 mL of contrast, the catheter tip was to the right of the midline at L1–2 and pointing caudally. The initial flow of contrast was seen to spread rapidly and to preferentially fill the right side of the subdural space from T6–L4 (Fig. 5.3a). There was late and limited contrast spread on the left side, with a very faint column between T6 and L1 and very little contrast towards the midline. A characteristic sign of subdural contrast is the tadpole-like collection in small pockets surrounding the proximal portion of the nerve roots, with the tadpole's head lying medially, and the tail curving away laterally to a fine point (Fig. 5.3b, arrowed), representing contrast running between the arachnoid and dura to lymph spaces within the root ganglia, and within the perineural lymphatics.

The lateral view (Fig. 5.3c) shows only faint attenuated anterior and posterior columns of contrast (red arrows), with a small midline collection at T12–L1. The intervertebral foramina are empty (blue arrows).

5.2 Intradural injection

The three cases of extensive subdural injection with resulting high blocks just described[7,8] were in great contrast to

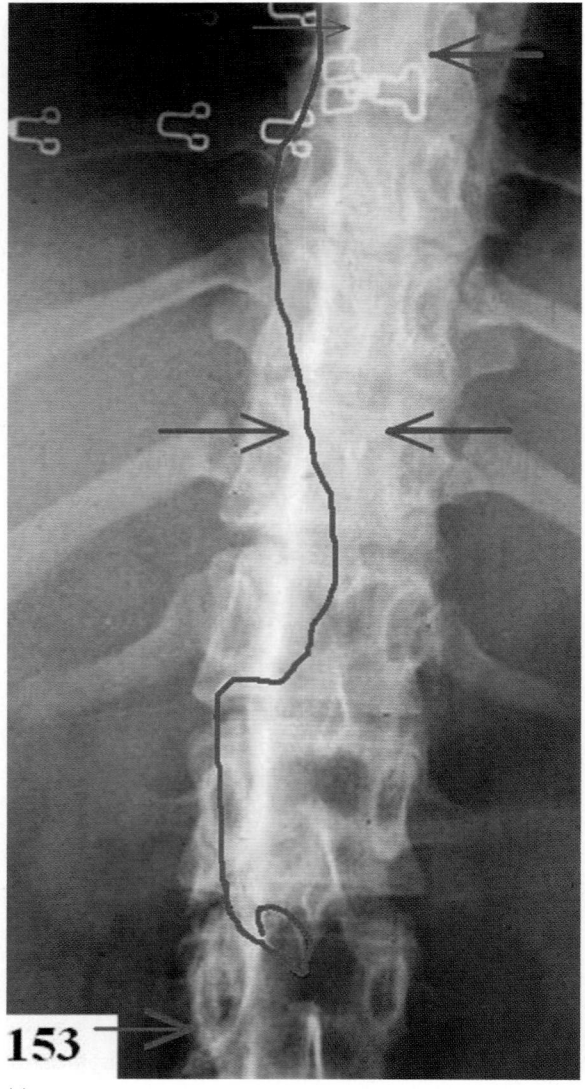

(a)

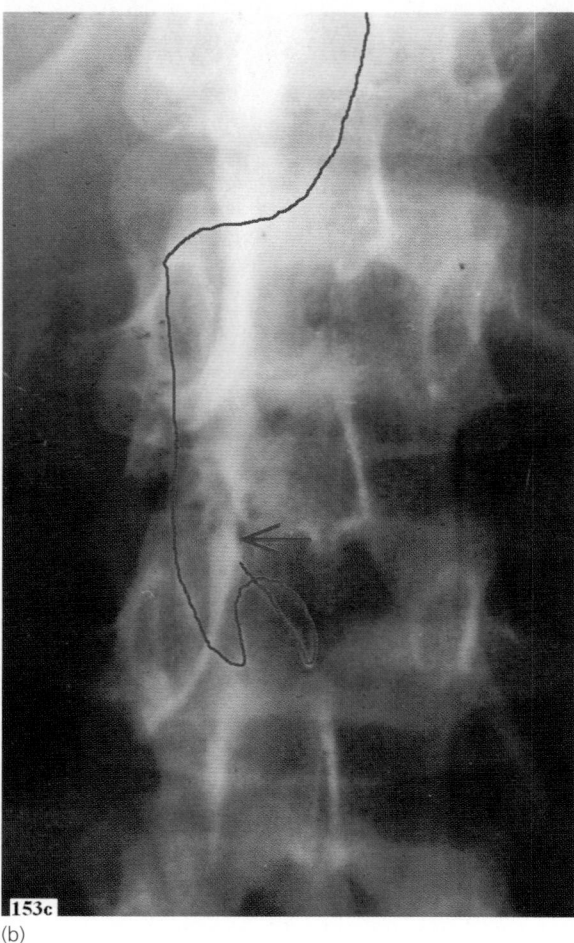

(b)

Fig. 5.3 (a) Anteroposterior (AP) epidurogram with predominantly right-sided column of subdural contrast from T6 to L4 (arrowed). The faint left-sided column is also indicated. (b) Detailed AP view of the same patient, to show the characteristic appearance of subdural contrast surrounding two adjacent spinal nerve roots. The outline of a posterior root ganglion is arrowed.

another 10 cases which had initially presented as cases of inadequate 'epidural' block in parturients.[12] These cases all showed a radiographic appearance unlike that seen following either epidural or subdural injection, with greatly limited vertical spread of contrast and the rapid formation of a dense mass of contrast.[12–14] We considered these cases, at that time, to be examples of 'atypical subdural injection' but later, to clarify the situation, we introduced the term 'intradural injection' based on our radiographic findings and the electron microscopy work of Reina *et al.*[15]

5.2.1 Radiographic appearances

5.2.1.1 The typical intradural image

The initial X-ray screening following contrast injection in these 10 patients showed the formation of a dense collection of localized contrast, which could not possibly be confused with either the thin, sometimes wispy, columns of

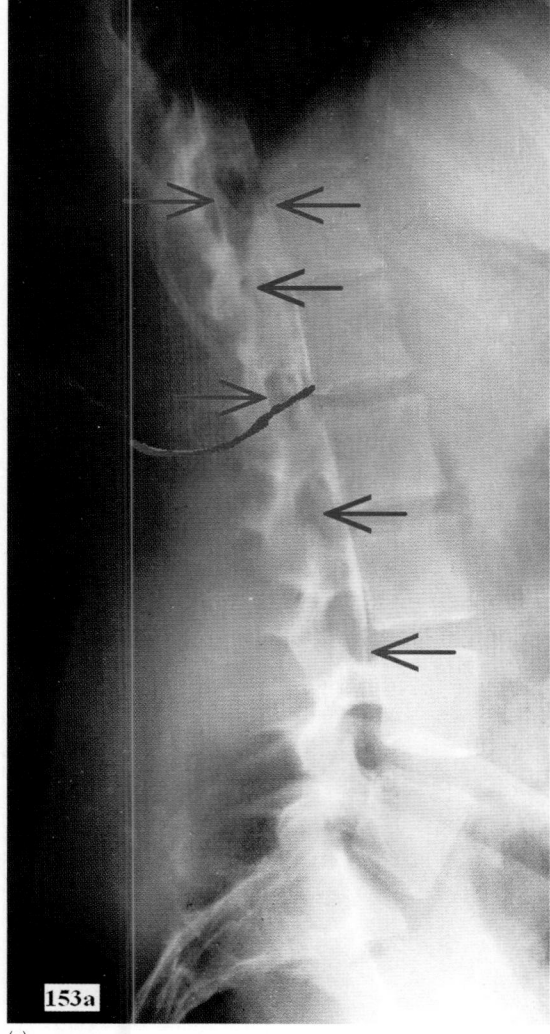

153a

(c)

● **Fig. 5.3** (Continued) (c) Lateral epidurogram showing faint anterior and posterior columns of subdural contrast (red arrows). There is only a small volume of midline contrast, with empty intervertebral foramina (blue arrows).

contrast that characterize true subdural injection (Figs 5.2 and 5.3), or epidural injection. In a typical AP view (Fig. 5.4a), the intradural collection appeared as a dense 'sausage-like' mass, extending over one to three vertebral segments, while a characteristic lateral view showed a mass that bulged anteriorly as the injected volume increased (Fig. 5.4b). Three-dimensional modelling based on the radiographs of this patient resulted in the image shown in Fig. 5.4c.

In five patients the injection of contrast produced low back pain, as the mass was seen to swell, and the procedure was ceased temporarily. As the pain recurred on resumption in three patients, injection was abandoned,

with the radiographs reflecting the reduced volume of contrast used (Figs 5.4 a,b, 5.5 and 5.6). In the other seven, a full (10–12 mL) dose of contrast was injected and the radiographic appearances, at this time, showed reasonable volumes of contrast escaping into the epidural space in five, into the subarachnoid space in one and the subdural space in another. A detailed description of three of these cases appears later (Case Histories 5.4, 5.5 and 5.6).

5.2.1.2 Intradural contrast escaping to the epidural space

In the five cases showing contrast flowing from the intradural space to the epidural space, the AP views demonstrated that the epidural contrast was unilateral in three (Figs 5.7a, 5.8a and 5.9a), with prominent foraminal spill in the first two. In the first case (Fig. 5.7a, p.52) the epidural contrast appears to have spread retrogradely around the epidural catheter to fill the left side of the epidural space from L5 to S2, with foraminal spill of contrast (blue arrows). The second case (Fig. 5.8, p.54) involved the same patient some 3 years later, and again there appears to be left-sided escape of contrast around the catheter to the epidural space anteriorly, as well as marked spill from the left L4 foramen (Fig. 5.8a, lower blue arrow). It is well known to radiologists that once a subdural space has been created, it may persist for many years, if not for ever, and be repeatedly entered by needles intended for myelography. The intradural space appears to act in a similar manner.

In the third case (Fig. 5.9a, p.55), faint right-sided epidural contrast (blue arrows) is seen lateral to the dense mass of intradural contrast (red arrows), but is more obvious in the lateral view (Fig. 5.9b). Bilateral epidural contrast filling was evident in the images from the fourth patient (Fig. 5.10a, p.56), which show a less dense mass of intradural contrast (red arrows) than the previous patient, but again the lateral view is diagnostic and faint epidural contrast is evident (blue arrows, Fig. 5.10b).

In all five patients the contrast injection, as seen on screening, appeared initially to create a dense intradural mass, before escaping into the epidural space, presumably around the outside of the epidural catheter, at least in the first four cases.

A different mechanism of spread seems likely in the remaining case (Fig. 5.11a, p.57), as the epidural contrast appeared only above T4, yet the catheter tip was at L3. Unfortunately interpretation of the contrast spread in this patient was hampered by poor-quality imaging.

CASE HISTORY 5.4:

HIGH INTRADURAL/EPIDURAL BLOCK

A 36-year-old undergoing her fifth elective caesarean section, following four successful epidural or CSE blocks,

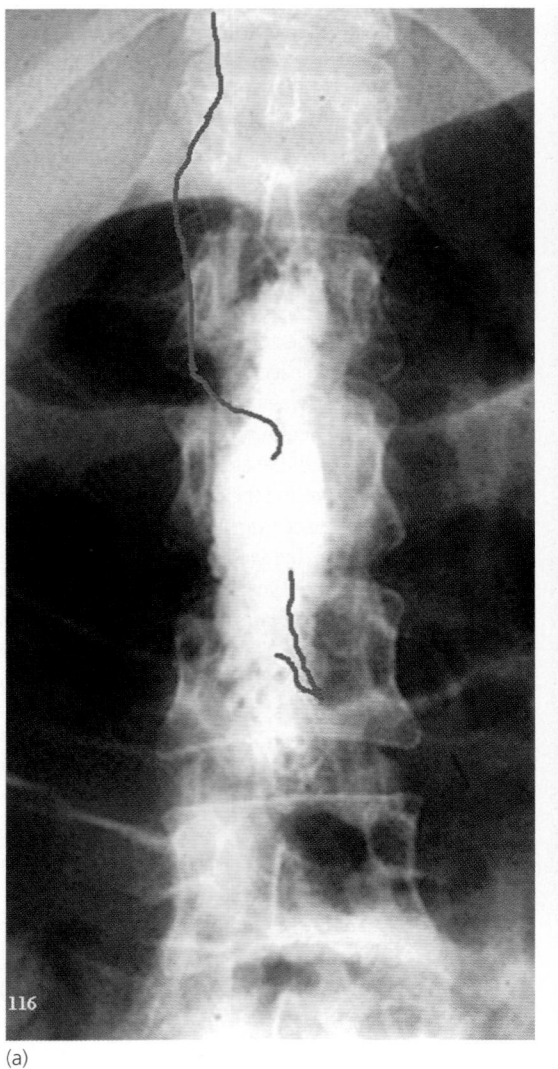

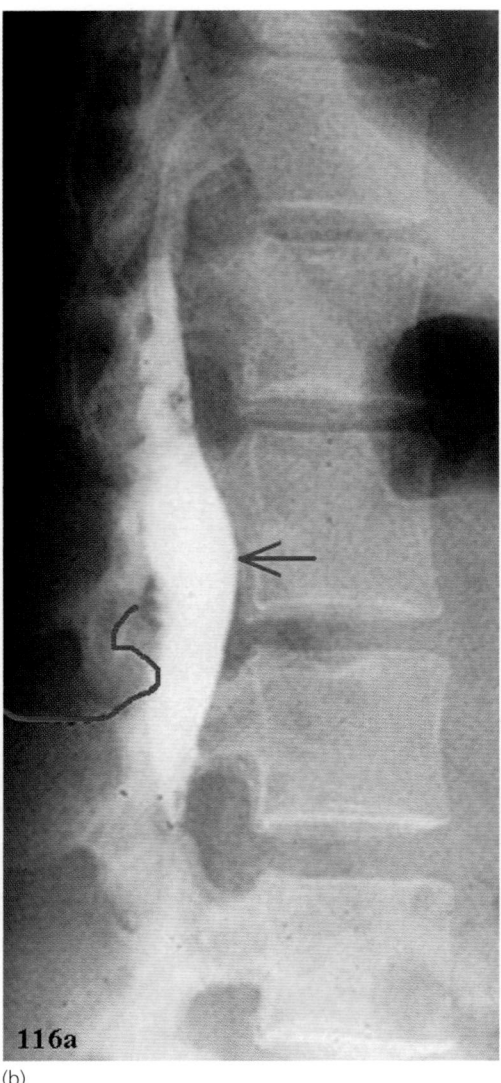

(a)   (b)

● **Fig. 5.4** (a) Anteroposterior (AP) epidurogram of thoracolumbar spine showing dense 'sausage-shaped' mass of intradural contrast. (b) Lateral radiograph with bulging mass of intradural contrast (arrowed) in the same patient.

received an apparently straightforward epidural insertion at L3–4. A dose of 17 mL ropivacaine 0.875% was given through the Tuohy needle in divided doses over 3 min, and it was noted that some of the injected local anaesthetic could be easily aspirated into the syringe during that time. When the syringe was disconnected 2–3 mL of the local anaesthetic (negative test for glucose) exited the hub of the Tuohy needle under some pressure. The procedure only resulted in a bilateral block to T6 after 20 min, and a further 10 mL of local anaesthetic was given through the epidural catheter. Ten minutes later, the block had reached T4 on pinprick testing, with immobile

legs (Bromage 3), and surgery was allowed to commence, but shortly afterwards the patient complained of numb hands, with slight difficulty in breathing and swallowing, together with mild hypotension. The block level was at T2 on pinprick testing, but started to regress over the next 20 min. Her further course was uneventful and she agreed to be investigated on the following day.

Epidurogram findings: **high intradural contrast, with epidural escape**

On AP screening, the tip of the epidural catheter was seen at L3 in the midline running rostrally (Fig. 5.11a, p.57).

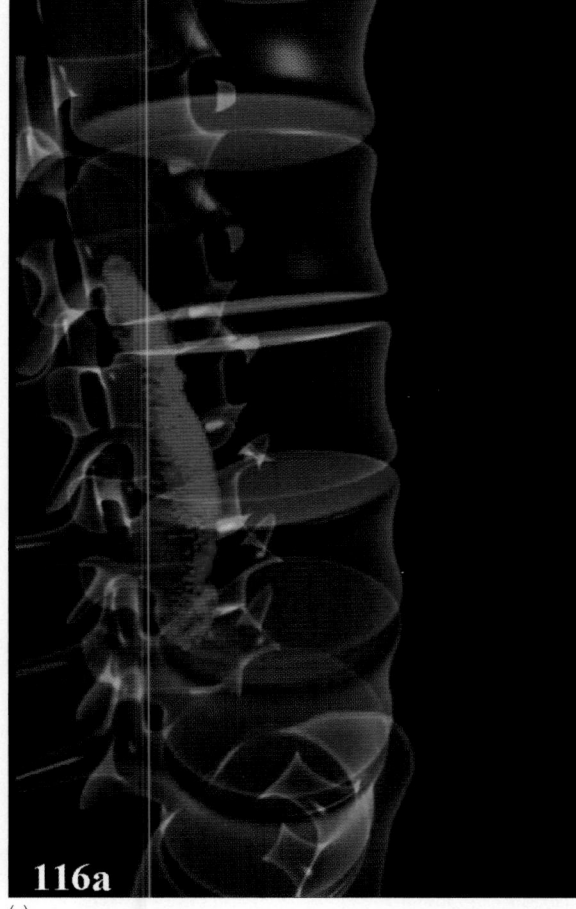

116a

(c)

● **Fig. 5.4** (Continued) (c) Three-dimensional modelling of the radiographs from the same patient (3D Studio Max). (Parts a and b reproduced from Collier CB. *Reg Anesth Pain Med* 2004; 29:45–51, with the kind permission of Lippincott Williams & Wilkins.)

A small collection of faint contrast (red arrows) appeared around the catheter tip, from L2 to L4, and was probably intradural, as it appeared to be related to a large dense mass of intradural contrast that extended from T6 to T12 and appeared to fill the whole width of the vertebral canal (Fig. 5.11b, red arrows). In both the AP radiographs, the outline of this mass is seen to be smooth, with its ends being rounded off, and there was no evidence of any emerging spinal nerves or nerve root structures. However, above this intradural mass, at T4, bilateral foraminal spill from the epidural space is faintly evident (Fig. 5.11b), although the radiograph is of poor quality and somewhat truncated.

Unfortunately, the lateral epidurogram (Fig. 5.11c) is also suboptimal, and does not show the position of the catheter tip, nor the high epidural contrast, but reveals extensive spread of a posterior mass of intradural contrast from T6 to T11, with several intermittently situated bulges (or, alternatively, indentations) positioned anteriorly, and apparently unrelated to the disc spaces. This 'scalloped' appearance had not been seen by us before, but Nir Hoftman (University of California Los Angeles Medical Center, USA) kindly supplied almost identical images (Fig. 5.12, p.59) following a complicated block for labour in a 23-year-old parturient, who had undergone several attempts at epidural needle insertion with the presence of cerebrospinal fluid (CSF) being repeatedly noted. The same 'sausage-like' mass appears in the AP view (Fig. 5.12a), and a similar scalloped appearance in the lateral view (Fig. 5.12b).

The cause of our patient's high block appears to have been escape of local anaesthetic from the intradural space to the epidural space. It is possible that retrograde flow around the epidural catheter could have occurred to such a high level, with any ascending epidural contrast being obscured by bowel shadows inferiorly and the dense mass of intradural contrast above. It would not be expected that the intradural solution could rupture through an intact dura in the thoracic spine, so unless there was a localized defect in the dura, the exact mechanism behind this high block remains open to speculation.

5.2.1.3 The typical lateral view of intradural contrast

An anterior bulging mass of contrast does appear to be characteristic of intradural injection. In some cases, there was only a single bulge in the lateral view (Figs 5.4b and 5.5b), in others there were two bulges (Fig. 5.9b), three bulges (Fig. 5.6b), or sometimes multiple swellings, at the thoracic level, as above (Figs 5.11c and 5.12b).

5.2.1.4 Intradural block and spina bifida occulta

An incidental radiographic finding has been the detection of spina bifida occulta (SBO) in 5 of our 10 patients with intradural block. This 50% incidence compares with our overall finding of SBO in 21% of parturients. There have been many attempts in the past to link the incidental finding of SBO to various medical conditions, with little success. So, while it is interesting to postulate on a possible connection between the finding of SBO and the presence of a congenital defect in the dura that might predispose to subdural injection, far more evidence is required, as discussed at the end of Chapter 8 (Section 8.5, p.109).

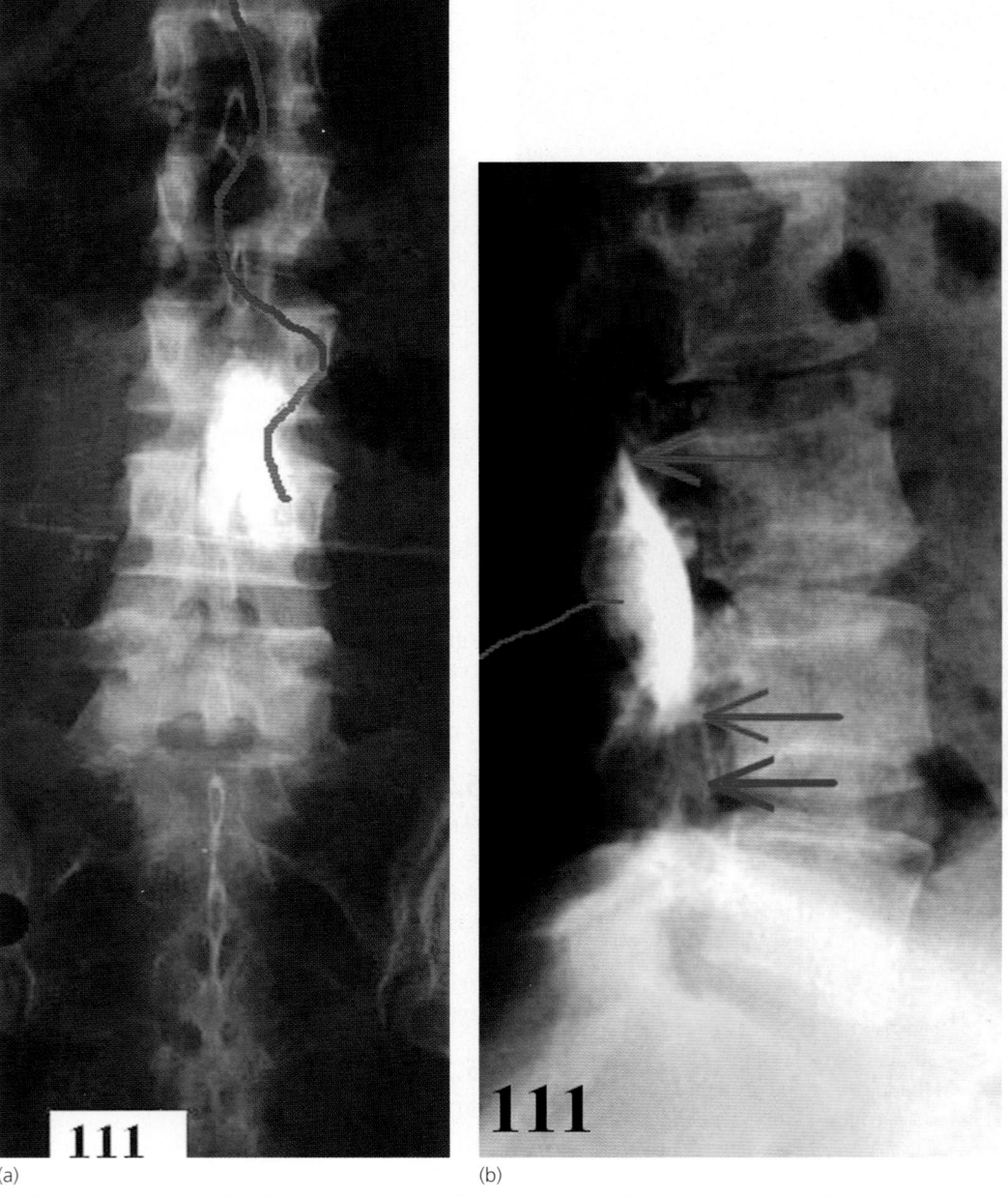

(a)   (b)

● **Fig. 5.5** (a) Anteroposterior (AP) radiograph showing small but dense mass of intradural contrast at L3–4, with no obvious epidural escape. (b) Lateral radiograph with bulging mass of intradural contrast (red arrows), between L3 and L4. Inferior to this, faint areas of contrast (blue arrow) probably indicate early epidural escape.

5.2.2 Clinical findings of intradural block

Of the 10 patients studied, four were in labour, two of them having undergone satisfactory epidural blocks for a previous delivery. One labouring patient progressed to emergency caesarean section and the remaining three had vaginal deliveries. The other six underwent repeat elective caesarean section under epidural block. The local anaesthetics used were bupivacaine, lidocaine or ropivacaine in appropriate

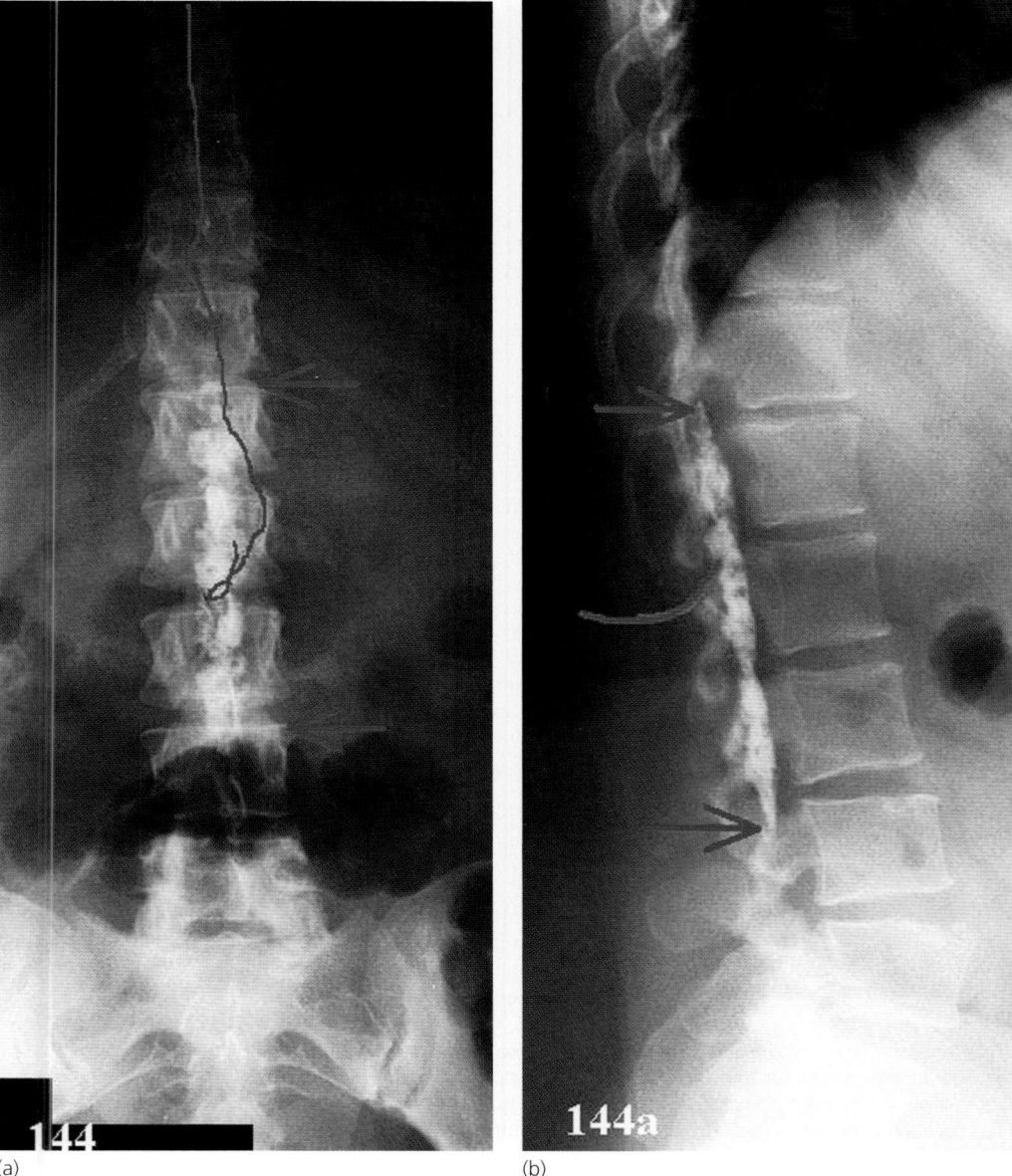

(a)   (b)

● **Fig. 5.6** (a) Anteroposterior (AP) radiograph showing a fairly dense narrow midline body of intradural contrast from L1 to L4 (arrowed), with a slightly irregular outline. (b) Lateral radiograph demonstrating a posterior mass of intradural contrast (arrowed) from L1 to L4.

concentrations, with adrenaline, fentanyl or pethidine added in some cases, at the choice of the individual anaesthetist.

The clinical features in these 10 patients with intradural block (Table 5.1, right column, p.41) are described below. These were quite different in many respects to those observed following subdural block (Table 5.1, left column):

1 In all cases, there had been an apparently straightforward and uneventful epidural needle and catheter insertion, mostly by highly experienced obstetric anaesthetists.

2 There was slow onset of an inadequate neuraxial block over 20–40 min.

3 The initial block was restricted in spread, and usually low and confined to a few adjacent dermatomes, which were often predominantly unilateral.

4 Following additional doses of local anaesthetic (10–20 mL), and the passage of 15–30 min, the blocks became clinically satisfactory in eight patients, presumably as a result of delayed epidural spread. Two of the six patients

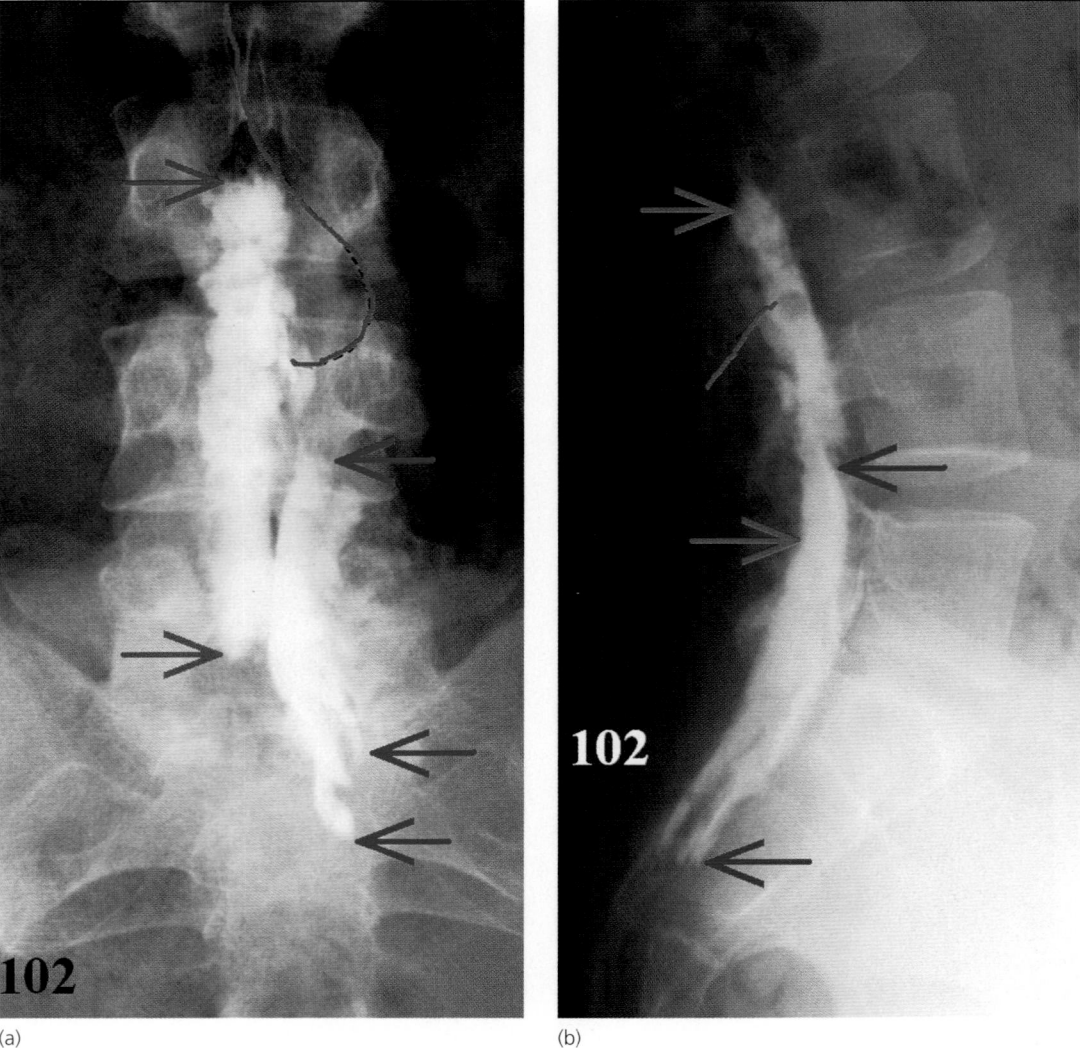

(a) (b)

Fig. 5.7 (a) Anteroposterior (AP) epidurogram revealing a dense central mass of intradural contrast (red arrows) from L3 to L5, with adjoining epidural contrast (blue arrows) from L4 to S1. L5 and S1 foraminal escape of contrast is seen (lower blue arrows). A minor degree of spina bifida occulta (SBO) is present at S1, but is not clearly visible in this image. (b) Lateral epidurogram showing overlapping collections of intradural (red arrows) and epidural contrast (blue arrows).

undergoing elective caesarean section briefly complained of slight abdominal discomfort during peritoneal mobilization, despite loss of sensation to pinprick to T4 preoperatively, but the outcome was considered satisfactory by all eight patients and no intravenous supplementation was required. In two labouring patients, top-up doses given more than 1 h after the original block resulted in a total spinal block in one and a high subdural block in the other (as described below). The other two labouring patients delivered vaginally with moderate, but short-lived, perineal pain being reported at delivery.

5 Five patients complained of atypical pain, either on epidural catheter insertion or during catheter injection of local anaesthetic or later contrast. The pain was usually short-lived, and just a dull ache in the back, but occasionally was more severe.

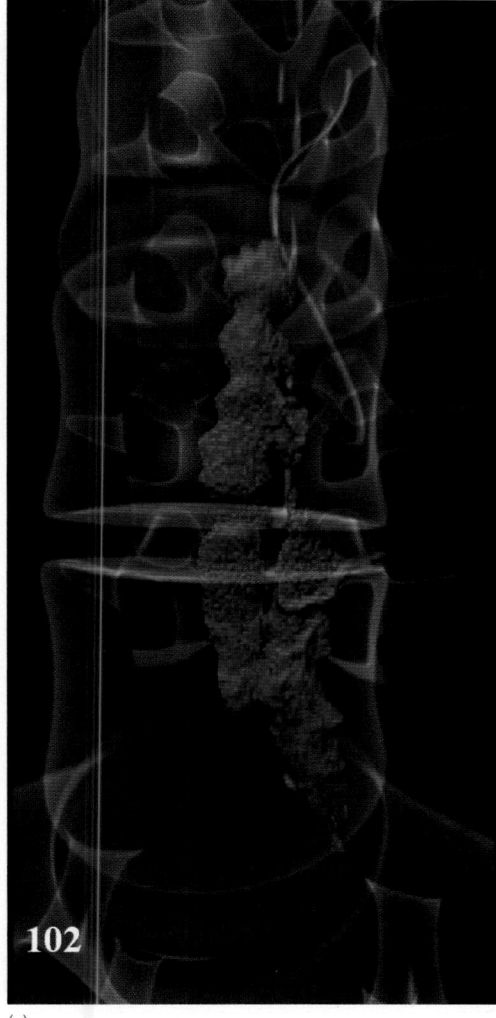

102

(c)

● **Fig. 5.7** (Continued) (c) Three-dimensional modelling of the radiographs from the same patient (3D Studio Max; the 'epidural' catheter is depicted in blue for clarity).

6 Following post-caesarean PCEA with injections of pethidine (30–50 mg in 10 mL solution, every 1–2 h as required) intense numbness developed in four patients, in a dermatomal distribution, affecting the legs, back or perineum, and persisted for 30–60 min.

CASE HISTORY 5.5:
TOTAL SPINAL BLOCK FOLLOWING INTRADURAL INJECTION

A total spinal block developed in a primiparous patient who had received an uneventful epidural block insertion in early labour with 16 mL 0.125% bupivacaine, although the pain relief was described as 'patchy', with a numb and heavy left leg (Bromage 2). When an emergency caesarean section was required 80 min later for foetal distress, a top-up dose of 10 mL lidocaine 2% with adrenaline was given, uneventfully, over 2 min following negative aspiration. A further 10 mL, given 2 min later, again after negative aspiration, resulted in the immediate collapse of the patient, with extreme hypotension and apnoea. Following resuscitation and general anaesthesia for surgery the patient awoke after 3 h and the block had totally regressed after 6 h. Cerebrospinal fluid could now be aspirated through the catheter and contrast injection was undertaken.

Epidurogram findings: combined intradural and subarachnoid contrast

Anteroposterior screening revealed the catheter tip to be behind the body of L3 in the midline, with a small dense mass of intradural contrast most prominent at L2–3 (Fig. 5.13a, p.60, red arrows) overlying the linear streaking of subarachnoid contrast. The characteristic horizontal upper level of subarachnoid contrast was at L1 (blue arrow), but moved freely with changes in patient position. The lateral view (Fig. 5.13b) shows the catheter entering a narrow mass of intradural contrast posteriorly, extending from L2 to L5 (red arrows), with faint subarachnoid linear streaking anteriorly (blue arrows). Recovery was straightforward, without the development of a postdural puncture headache.

Figure 5.17k (p.70) is an electron microscopy image (courtesy Professor M. A. Reina, Madrid, Spain) showing how an epidural catheter in the intradural space might migrate into the subarachnoid space.

CASE HISTORY 5.6:
HIGH SUBDURAL BLOCK, FOLLOWING INTRADURAL INJECTION

A primiparous patient presented for epidural block in labour and a dose of 14 mL bupivacaine 0.25% with adrenaline was injected over 5 min. Good analgesia resulted, with a sensory block extending from T8 to L4 and mild hypotension.

Three hours later a top-up was requested and 12 mL of the same solution was injected over 2 min following negative aspiration. Hypotension (90/50 mmHg) occurred after 15 min. At 25 min, the patient complained of numbness of her whole body up to the clavicles, followed

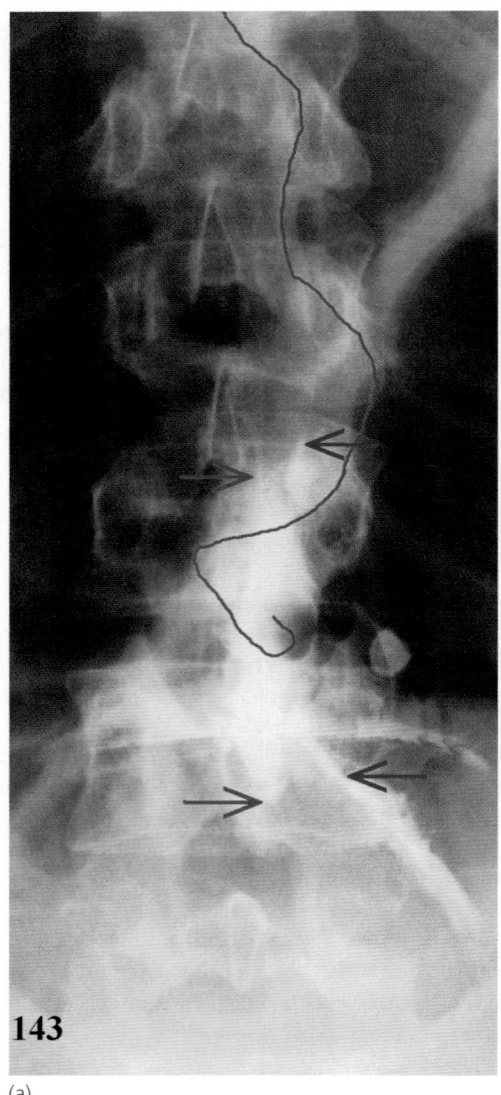

(a)

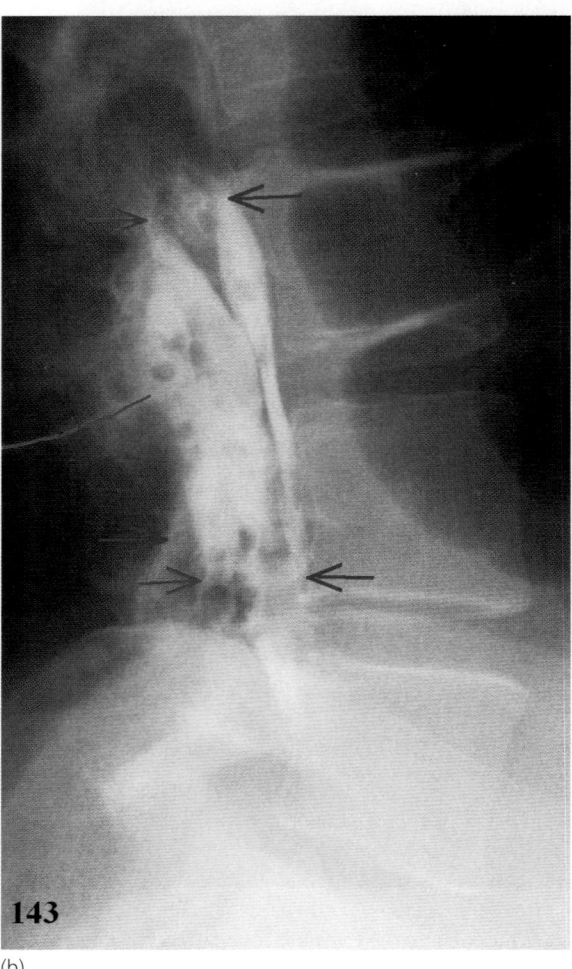

(b)

● **Fig. 5.8** (a) Anteroposterior (AP) epidurogram in the same patient as Fig. 5.7, 3 years later. This time the intradural contrast (red arrows) extends from L3 to L4, with the epidural escape at the same levels, with pronounced spill at L4 on the left (lower blue arrow). Again, the spina bifida occulta (SBO) is not clearly seen. (b) Lateral radiograph with dense intradural contrast between L3 and L4 posteriorly (red arrows) with epidural contrast anteriorly (blue arrows) and L4 root spill (blue arrow).

by a feeling of heaviness in her left arm, both legs, chest and perineum. Sensory testing revealed numbness to pinprick up to C3 on the left and T2 on the right. There was slight weakness of the left hand, and the legs were immobile (Bromage 3). There were no pupillary changes. The respiration was noted to be slightly uncoordinated. The blood pressure again responded to fluid loading, and remained stable (135/80) thereafter. A forceps delivery

was undertaken satisfactorily for foetal bradycardia and the block had completely regressed after a total of 4 h.

Epidurogram findings: combined intradural and subdural contrast

Contrast injection (8 mL) was performed 4 h later and the initial AP screening showed the catheter tip at L3 in the midline, with a low 'sausage-like' mass of intradural

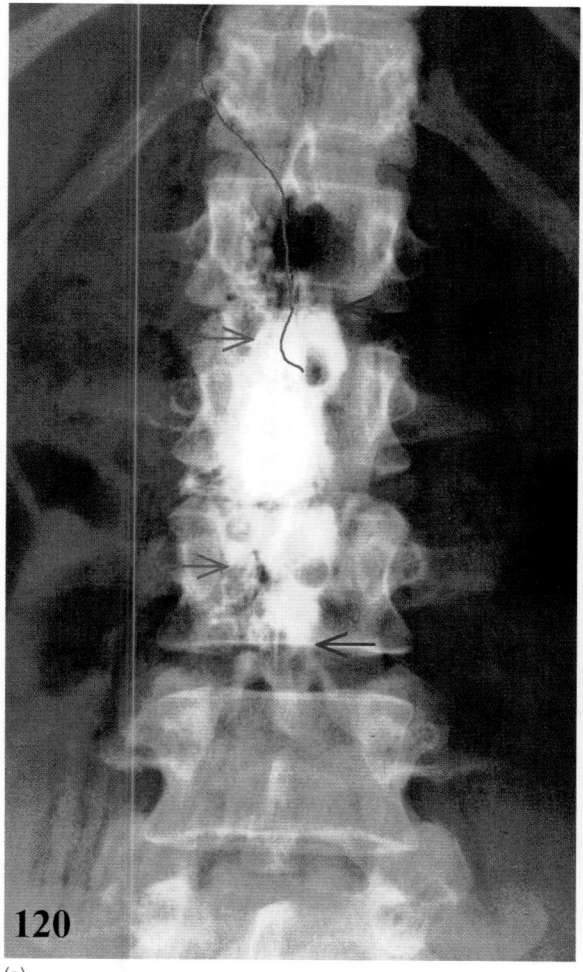

(a)

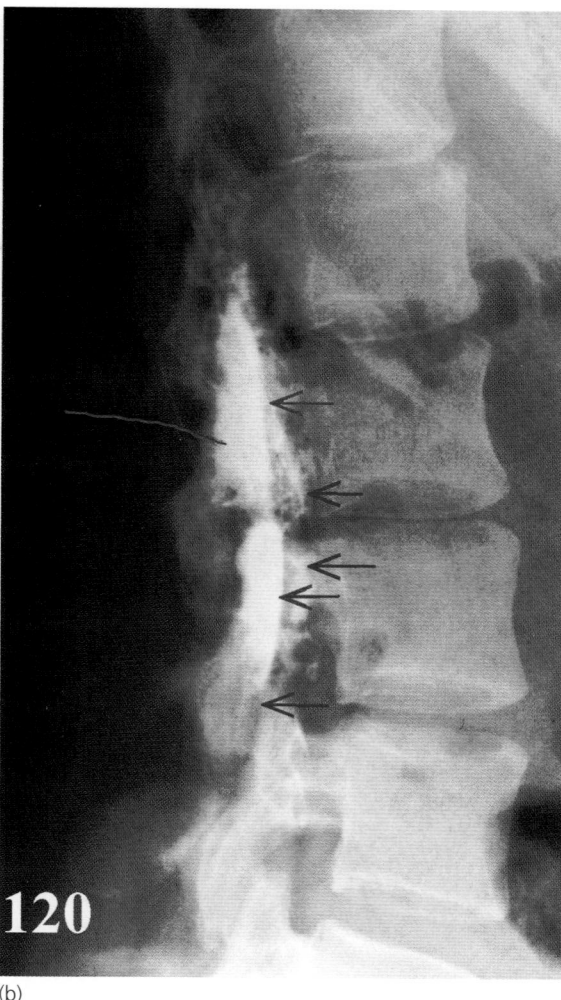

(b)

● **Fig. 5.9** (a) Anteroposterior (AP) epidurogram with a small but dense central mass of intradural contrast between L1 and L3 (red arrows), with a small volume of escaping epidural contrast on the right side at the same levels (blue arrows). (b) Lateral epidurogram showing two bulging masses of intradural contrast (red arrows). A small volume of epidural contrast lies anteriorly (blue arrows).

contrast from L3-S1 (red arrows, Fig. 5.14a, p.61), which, in the lateral view, is seen to be bulging anteriorly into the vertebral canal (red arrow, Fig. 5.14c). The AP screening then revealed the cephalad spread of subdural contrast from L3 to T8 bilaterally (blue arrows, Fig. 5.14a) with limited nerve root contrast filling from L4 upwards. There is some overlap between the masses of intradural and subdural contrast, with no clear distinction apparent. The caudal end of the mass of intradural contrast is

shown in a magnified view in Fig. 5.14b, as it approaches a spina bifida occulta defect at S1 (yellow arrow).

The upper part of the lateral epidurogram shows marked anterior and posterior columns of contrast – the 'railroad track' appearance (blue arrows, Fig. 5.14c) – with empty intervertebral foramina between, being the typical appearance of a subdural block,[7] which is also modelled in Fig. 5.14d. Recovery was uneventful.

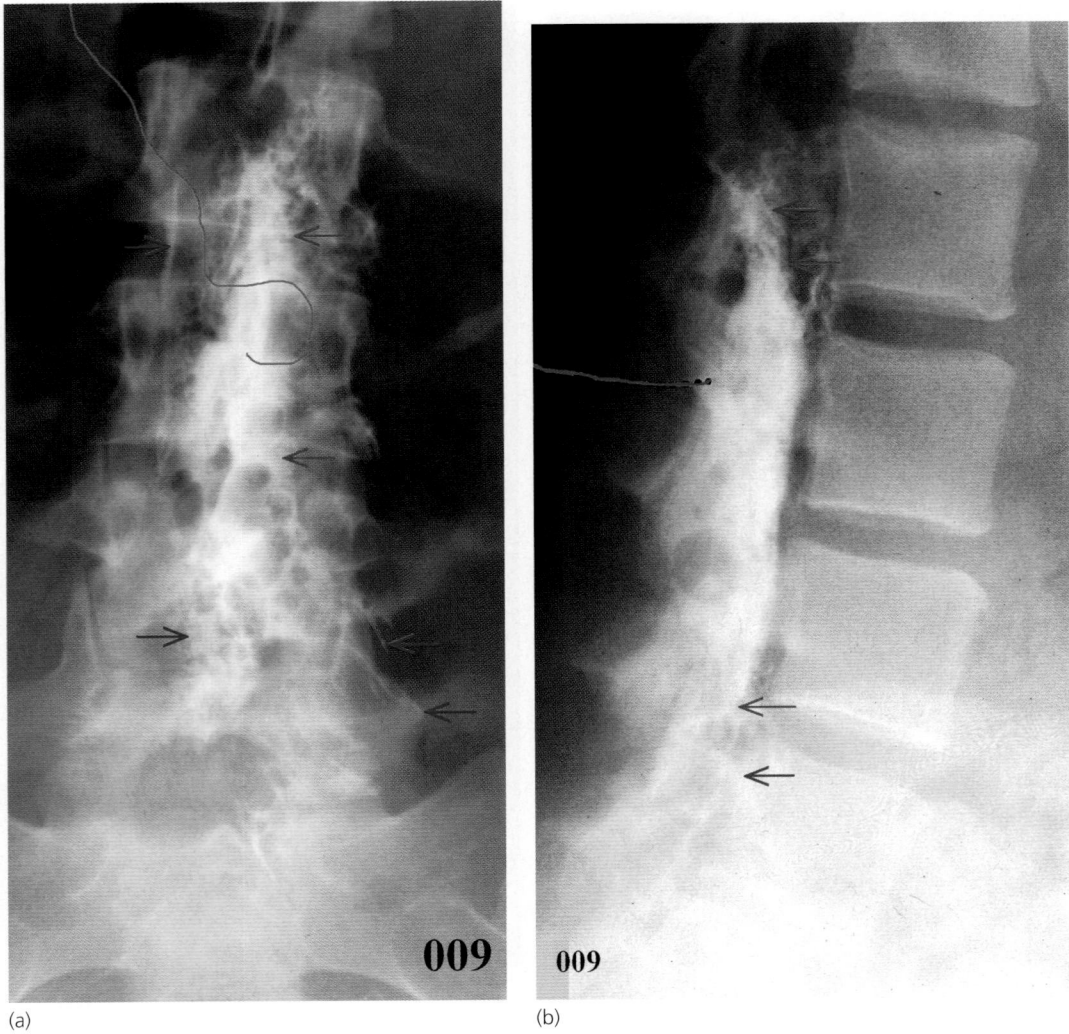

(a)   (b)

● **Fig. 5.10** (a) Anteroposterior (AP) radiograph revealing a small dense central mass of intradural contrast at L3–4 (red arrows) with bilateral escaping epidural contrast between L2 and L5 (blue arrows). Spina bifida occulta (SBO) is evident at S1. (b) Lateral epidurogram with a dense posterior mass of intradural contrast from L2 to L5 (red arrows), with patchy escaping epidural contrast above and below (blue arrows).

5.3 Discussion

5.3.1 Subdural/intradural anatomy

The subdural space is well known to anaesthetists and radiologists as a possible site of misplacement of epidural and spinal needles and catheters, but until recently, little detail of the microscopic anatomy of the region was known, and the published radiographic images often appeared to be conflicting. For example, Fig. 5.2a (p.44) shows a typical appearance of extensive thin wispy parallel columns of contrast following a high subdural block (to T2), whereas other published images, also titled

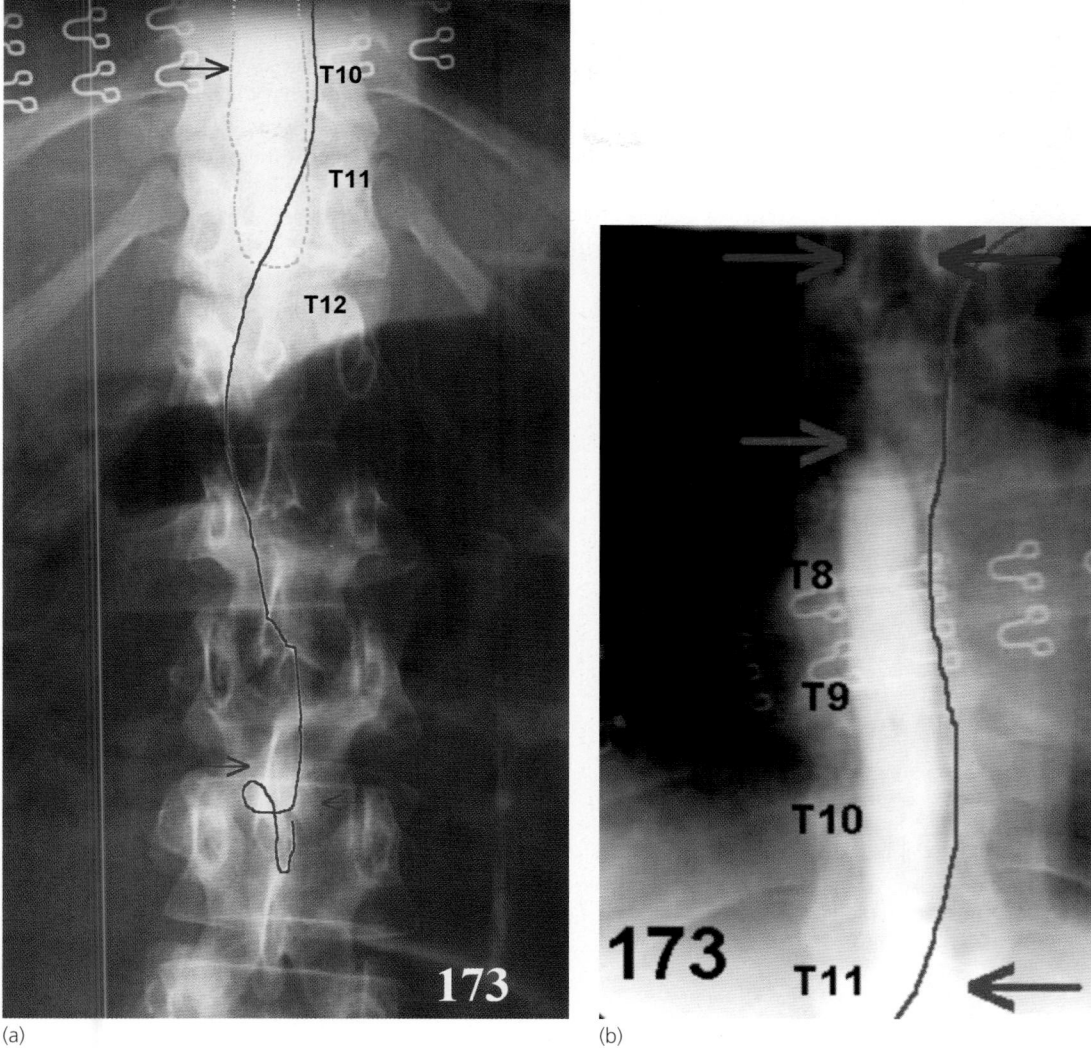

(a)   (b)

● **Fig. 5.11** (a) Anteroposterior (AP) epidurogram (lower half only). A faint collection of intradural contrast surrounds the catheter tip at L3 (red arrows), while the main body of dense intradural contrast is outlined (in green, with a blue arrow) and is seen to start at T12 and disappear off the film at T9 as it spreads to T6 (next image). (b) An AP epidurogram (upper half only) showing the upward extension of the dense column of intradural contrast to T6 (red arrows), with escaping epidural contrast appearing bilaterally at the level of the T4 foramina (blue arrows).

'subdural injection' (Fig. 5.15, p.63),[16] have shown a very different appearance, with a dense 'sausage-like' mass of contrast in the AP view, bulging towards the subarachnoid space in the lateral view, very similar to our images of intradural block. It is difficult to reconcile these two entirely different sets of images with a single diagnosis of 'subdural injection', and the presence of two separate spaces, probably adjacent to one another, has to be considered.

With regard to the anatomy, recent work has shown that the subdural space is not a potential space as previously thought, but is only produced as a result of trauma and tissue damage creating a cleft within the meninges.[15–18] Reina *et al*.[15] have reported that the arachnoid mater has a compact

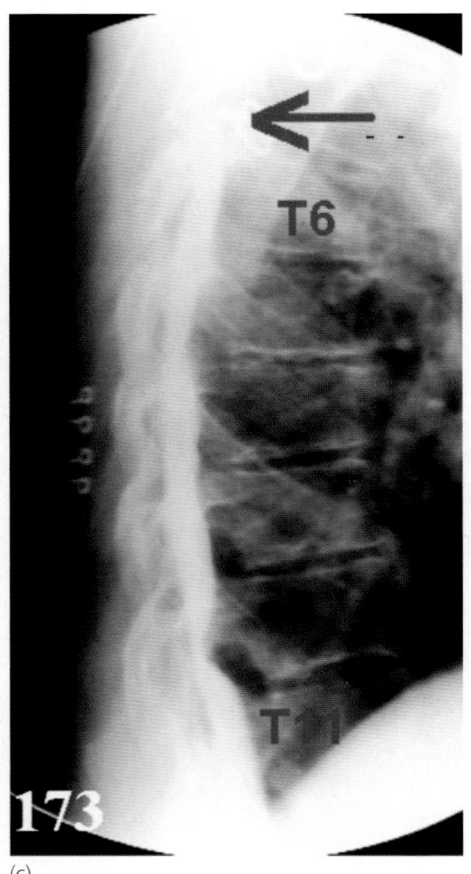

(c)

● **Fig. 5.11** (Continued) (c) Lateral epidurogram showing the upward extension of a dense posterior column of intradural contrast from T12 to T6 (red arrows), with multiple bulges at varying positions.

laminar portion that is adjacent to the innermost layers of the dura, and a trabeculated portion that spreads like a spider's web to the pia mater coating the spinal cord and nerve roots (Fig. 5.16a, p.64, left side). Between the laminar arachnoid portion and the inner surface of the dura they found a cellular interface they called the dura–arachnoid interface or subdural compartment. This region is composed of neurothelial cells surrounded by an amorphous substance (Fig. 5.16a, right side). There was no subdural space in non-traumatized tissues, but they found that a subdural space could be created (Fig. 5.16b) if the neurothelial cells broke up as a result of pressure exerted by mechanical forces, air or fluid injection. This produced fissures within the

amorphous substance of the interface. Fissures could readily expand towards weaker areas, particularly laterally where the amorphous substance is more prolific.[15] These fissures may combine to form what the authors called the primary subdural space (Fig. 5.16a, right side), which may be relatively short or extend to almost the whole length of the vertebral column and occasionally into the cranial cavity. Injection of routine epidural doses of local anaesthetic into this primary subdural space appears to result in the symptoms and signs of an extensive block that we recognize clinically as subdural block, with apnoea and unconsciousness in the most severe cases.

A number of secondary subdural spaces were also described by Reina *et al.*[15] as running parallel to the primary space (I in Fig. 5.17a, p.65). Some of the secondary spaces were more superficial than the primary space, being found encroaching into the substance of the dura. In this region, the collagen fibres that are the major component of the dura are fairly sparsely arranged. It appears possible that injection of contrast into this area, or secondary subdural space, could produce the encapsulated swelling mass with anterior ballooning of the remaining thin layers of the dura and the arachnoid, as seen in our radiographs and those of others.[16] We have preferred to call this area the 'intradural' space, rather than the secondary subdural space, to clearly distinguish it from the primary subdural space, a distinction that has caused some confusion in the past.

Professor M. A. Reina has kindly provided some of his electron microscopy images, produced following cadaver dissection. He noted that the thickness of the dura was approximately 250–400 μm. Samples of dura at the level of the dural sac showed it to be composed of approximately 80 bundles of fibres with a well-defined morphology. These bundles, which were arranged in concentric rings or laminae (Fig. 5.17b), were approximately 4–6 μm in diameter and composed of 10–12 collagen fibres and a few elastic fibres (Fig. 5.17c). Each lamina extended along the entire circumference of the sac (Fig. 5.17b). Variations in laminar thickness were caused by the number of collagen fibres that constituted each lamina. Dural laminae from samples that had been previously dehydrated could become detached from one another, keeping their shape unaltered while allowing an artefactual intradural space to develop (Fig. 5.17c–e). We believe that the intradural space, whether artefactual or produced by needle/catheter insertion, is

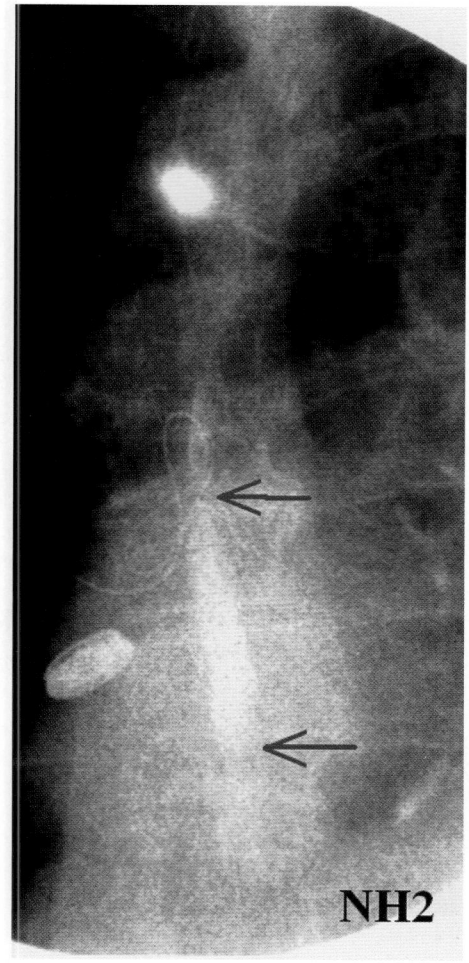

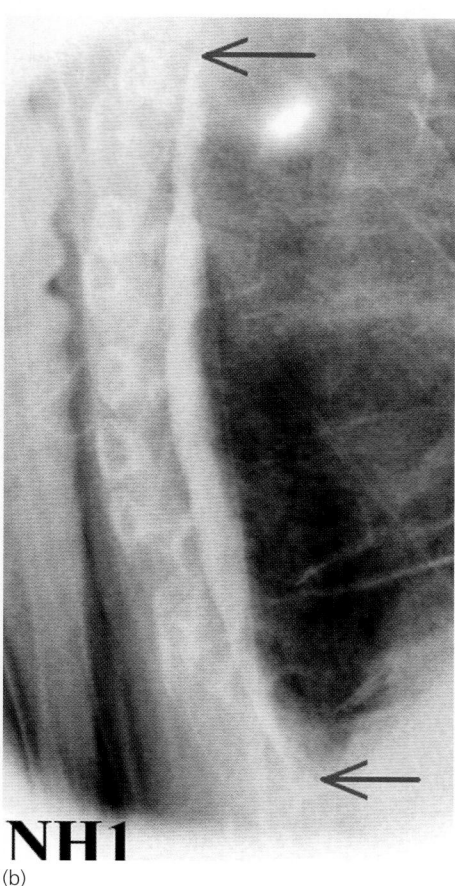

● **Fig. 5.12** (a) Anteroposterior (AP) radiograph following contrast injection in a 23-year-old parturient who suffered a dural puncture during attempted epidural block. A dense central mass of intradural contrast is seen in the mid-thoracic spine, similar to Fig. 5.10b, p.56. (b) Lateral radiograph in the same patient, showing a dense posterior column of intradural contrast, in the mid-thoracic spine (red arrows) with multiple bulges (or indentations) at varying positions, almost identical to Fig. 5.11c. (Images kindly supplied by Nir Hoftman, University of California Los Angeles Medical Center, USA.)

formed by dural delamination rather than tearing of the dural layers themselves.[19] The intradural space is concentric and parallel to the dural layers.

The intradural, or fourth space, as well as subdural spaces, are clearly seen in Fig. 5.17f,g. Reina was also able to introduce an epidural catheter into a subdural space (Fig. 5.17h) and an intradural space (Fig. 5.17i). Following removal of the intradural catheter, a cavity is left behind

(Fig. 5.17j). Figure 5.17k shows how an intradural catheter might migrate into the subarachnoid space, as in Case History 5.5, above. Once again, a cavity remains following catheter removal (Fig. 5.17l).

Filling of the intradural space is demonstrated in Fig. 5.18a (p.71). Figure 5.18 depicts stylized anatomical models of contrast injection, based on our epidurograms and further electron microscopy images of the dura–arachnoid

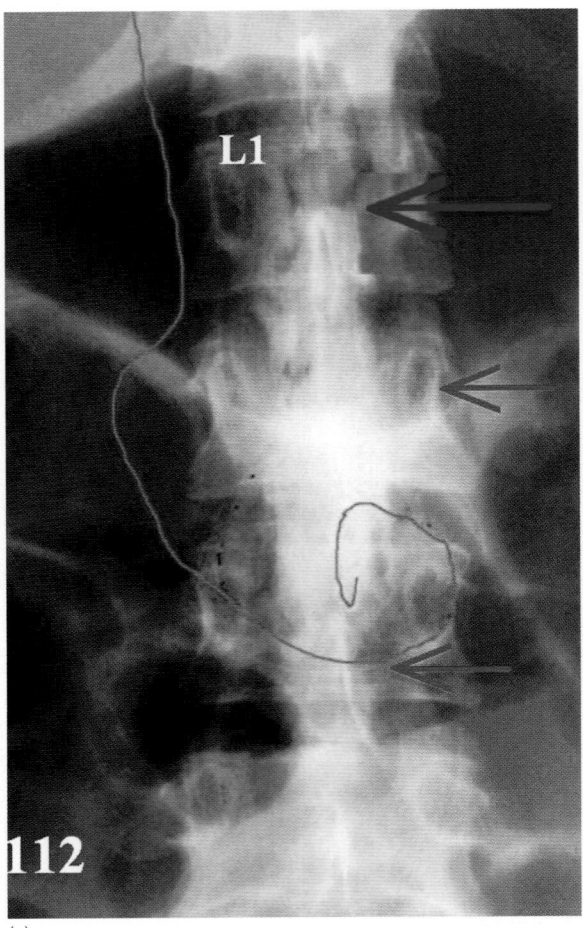

(a)

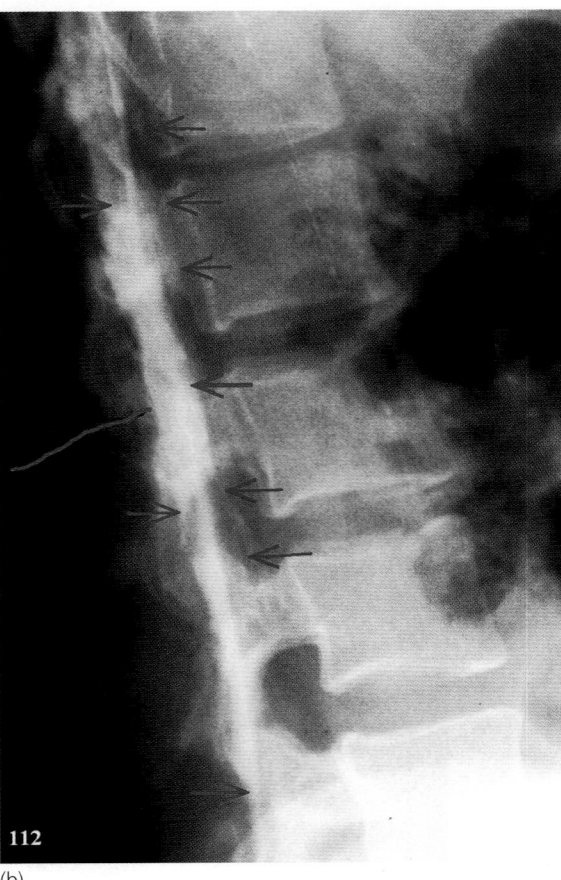

(b)

● **Fig. 5.13** (a) Anteroposterior (AP) epidurogram showing a dense mass of intradural contrast at L2–3 (red arrows) surrounding the catheter tip, and the horizontal upper level of a column of subarachnoid contrast (blue arrow). (b) Lateral radiograph with posterior intradural contrast from L2 to L4 (red arrows) and the faint linear streaking of subarachnoid contrast anteriorly (blue arrows).

interface. Adobe Photoshop (Adobe Systems, Chatswood, NSW, Australia) and Autodesk Combustion (Autodesk, Inc., San Rafael, CA, USA) programs were used to build up the complete pictures (for moving images please see the accompanying website).

Further injection may result in retrograde escape of some of the solution to the epidural space around the outside of the catheter (Fig. 5.18b), or rupture anteriorly through the remaining layers of the dura, to allow access to the subdural space (Fig. 5.18c). Occasionally the arachnoid is also disrupted, allowing entry to the subarachnoid space (Fig. 5.18d). The latter occurrence has been suggested as a possibility by several workers over recent years,[1,20] but proof has not previously been forthcoming. It has to be assumed, in

all these situations, that the spread of radiographic contrast reflects that of the prior local anaesthetic.

In summary, the radiographic appearances of an intradural injection are entirely different from that seen following a true subdural block but, unfortunately, they have often been generically labelled as 'subdural' by many radiologists and anaesthetists in the past.[4,16]

5.3.2 Clinical findings of subdural/intradural block

The clinical picture of an intradural block is quite different from that of a subdural block, at least initially, as intradural blocks present as a failed or inadequate block,

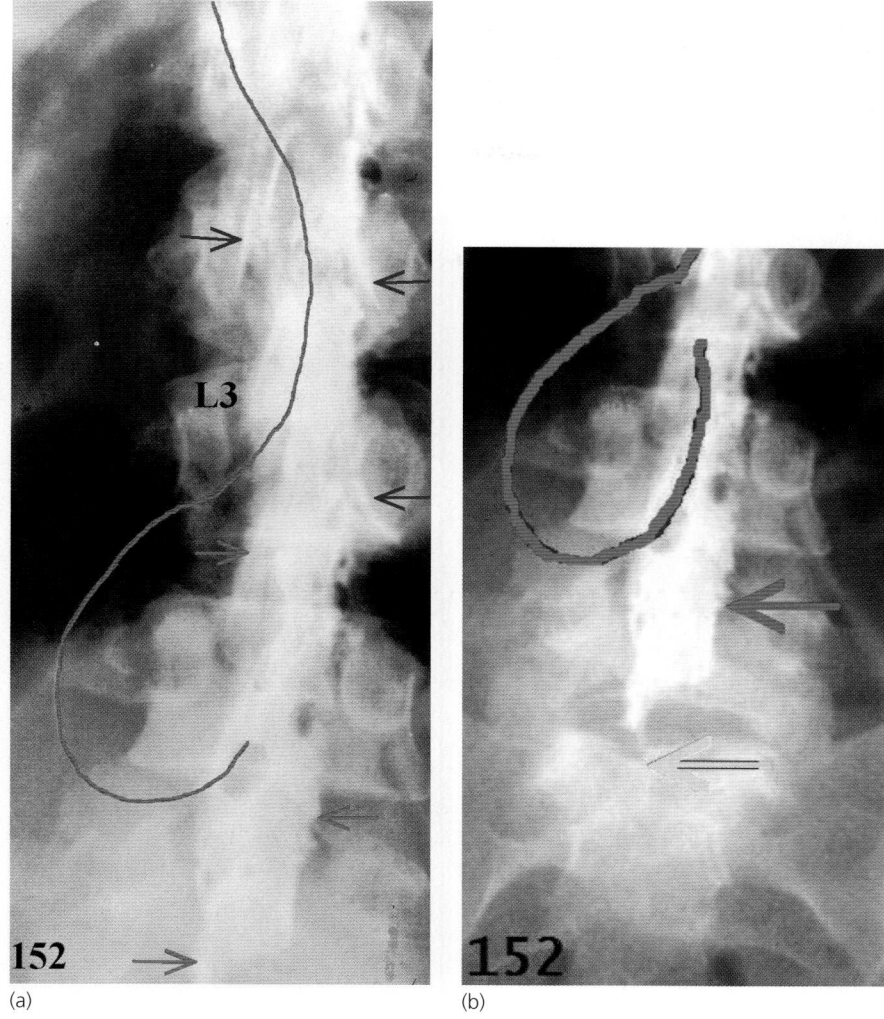

Fig. 5.14 (a) Anteroposterior (AP) radiograph of thoracolumbar spine showing a mass of intradural contrast between L3 and S1 (red arrows) merging above with subdural contrast, which outlines the L2–3 and L3–4 nerve roots (blue arrows). (b) An AP close-up view of the lower lumbar and sacral area of the same patient, showing the lower end of the intradural contrast down to L5 (red arrow) and spina bifida occulta at S1 (yellow arrow).

not an extended block. Some degree of inadequacy may be overlooked in the labouring patient, but becomes very obvious on block testing prior to caesarean section. Most anaesthetists faced with an inadequate block would inject an additional volume of local anaesthetic. This eventually proved successful in most of our patients, probably as a result of retrograde spread of solution to the epidural space. However, some caution is required, bearing in mind our two patients who developed high blocks of delayed onset.

The other unusual clinical findings with intradural block were the pain developed by some patients during 'epidural' catheter insertion and with the injection of local anaesthetic or contrast medium, as well as the numbness following pethidine injection postoperatively in others. The pain may be explained by the anterior swelling of the intradural mass coming into contact with the nerve roots of the cauda equina, or the spinal cord, at higher levels, as the collection may extend over half the AP diameter of the vertebral canal. The numbness almost certainly resulted from the restricted

61

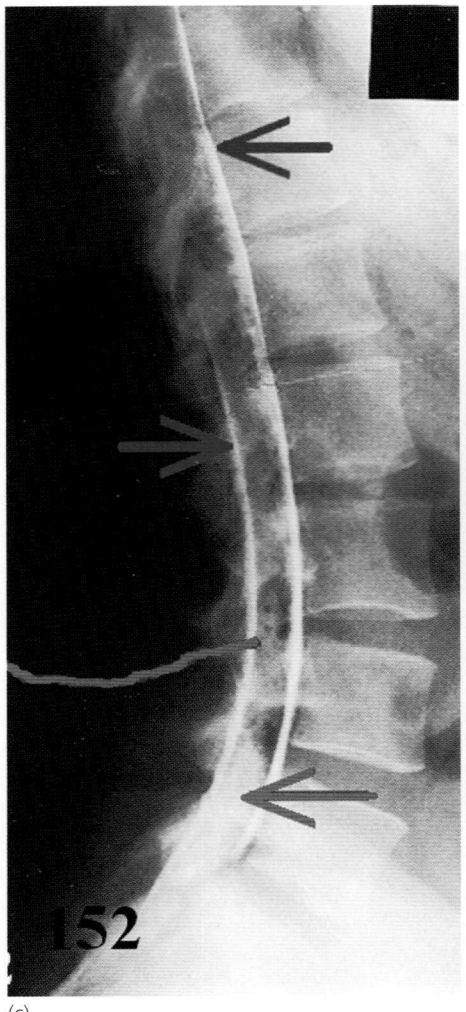

(c)

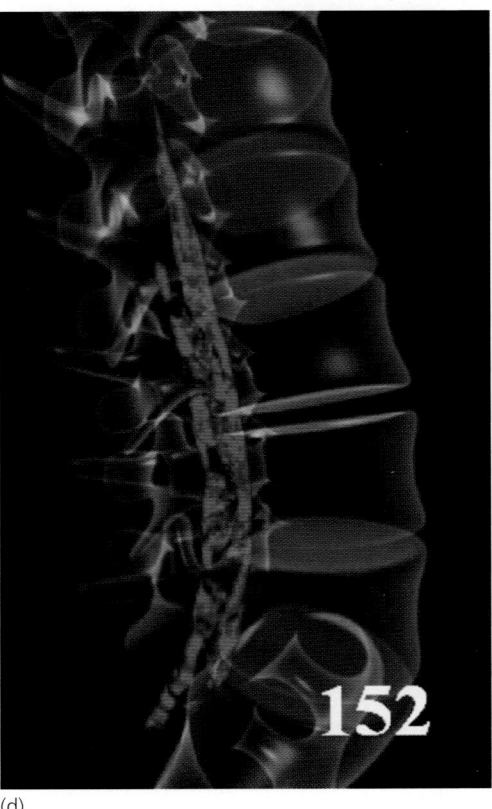

(d)

● **Fig. 5.14** (Continued) (c) Lateral view of thoracolumbar spine showing mass of intradural contrast from L3 to S1 (red arrow) and 'railroad tracks' of subdural contrast (blue arrows) above. (d) Three-dimensional modelling of the radiographs from the same patient (3D Studio Max), showing merging masses of intradural contrast below and subdural contrast above. (Parts a and c reproduced from Collier CB. *Anaesth Intens Care* 1992; 20:215–232 with the kind permission of The Australian Society of Anaesthetists Ltd.)

vertical spread of intradural pethidine, allowing a high localized concentration to accumulate in the dorsal columns of the spinal cord, accentuating the local anaesthetic properties of this opioid.

The finding of a total spinal block, with CSF aspiration, developing after a presumed initial intradural injection, may account for some of the many unexplained mysteries of the past, when there were reports of patients collapsing following a top-up dose some time, often many hours,

after the establishment of a clinically satisfactory epidural block.[20–23] Such cases were, at the time, either attributed to catheter migration or multicompartment block.

5.3.3 Incidence of subdural/intradural block

Our exact incidence of intradural injection is unknown, as we have only recently started specifically investigating

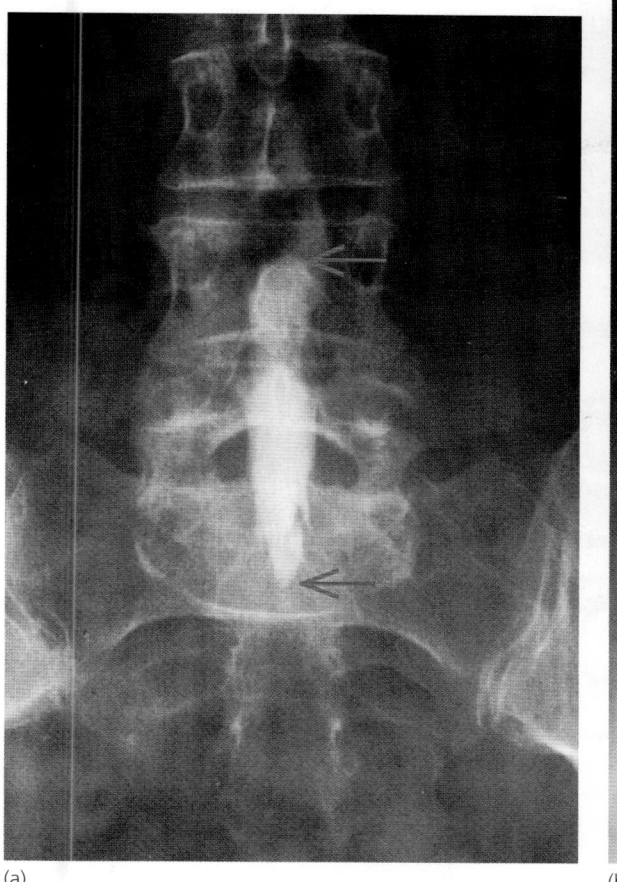 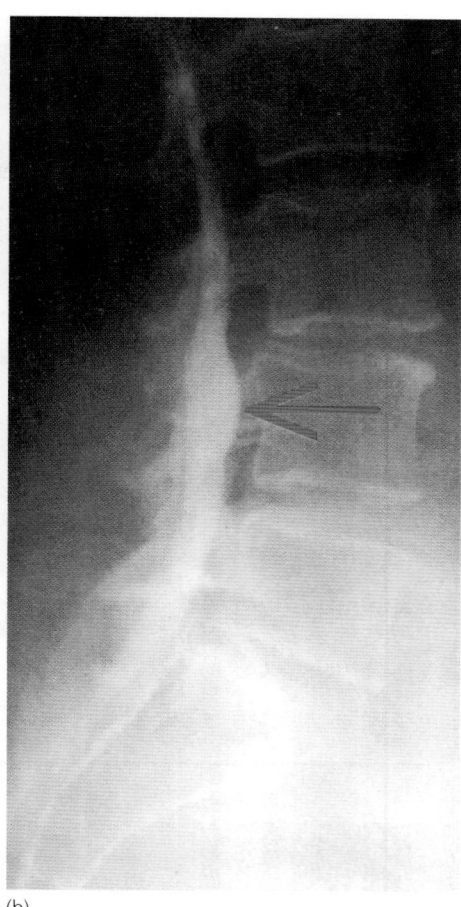

(a)   (b)

● **Fig. 5.15** (a) A published image labelled 'Anteroposterior (AP) radiograph of the lumbar spine with subdural contrast media' (arrowed). (b) A published image labelled 'Lateral radiograph of the lumbar spine with subdural contrast media' (arrowed). (Figures modified from Ajar AH, Rathmell JP, Mukherji SK. The subdural compartment. *Regional Anesthesia and Pain Medicine* 2002; 27:72–76, with permission.)

blocks of slow onset, which required additional doses of local anaesthetic, as well as all cases of late subarachnoid block with CSF aspiration. Previously, we declined to investigate many of the latter cases that were referred to us in the mistaken belief that the catheter had to be entirely intrathecal, and that no useful data would be forthcoming.

The incidence of intradural block, in our hands, appears to be around 1 in 500 attempted lumbar epidural blocks in parturients, which is higher than that of subdural block of approximately 1 in 3000 obstetric cases, but many cases will go unrecognized. Whatever the incidence of intradural block, it will remain only a rare cause of a failed or inadequate block. More common causes are escape of an epidural catheter through an intervertebral foramen, an obstructive septum and bony anomalies, such as scoliosis, or previous spinal surgery.[22]

5.3.4 Aetiology of intradural block

The aetiology of intradural injection is unknown, but one explanation may possibly involve the presence of scarring or adhesions in the epidural space and dura–arachnoid following previous catheter insertion or blood-patching. Long-term epidural catheter use is known to be associated with fibrosis in the epidural space[24]. It may be relevant that

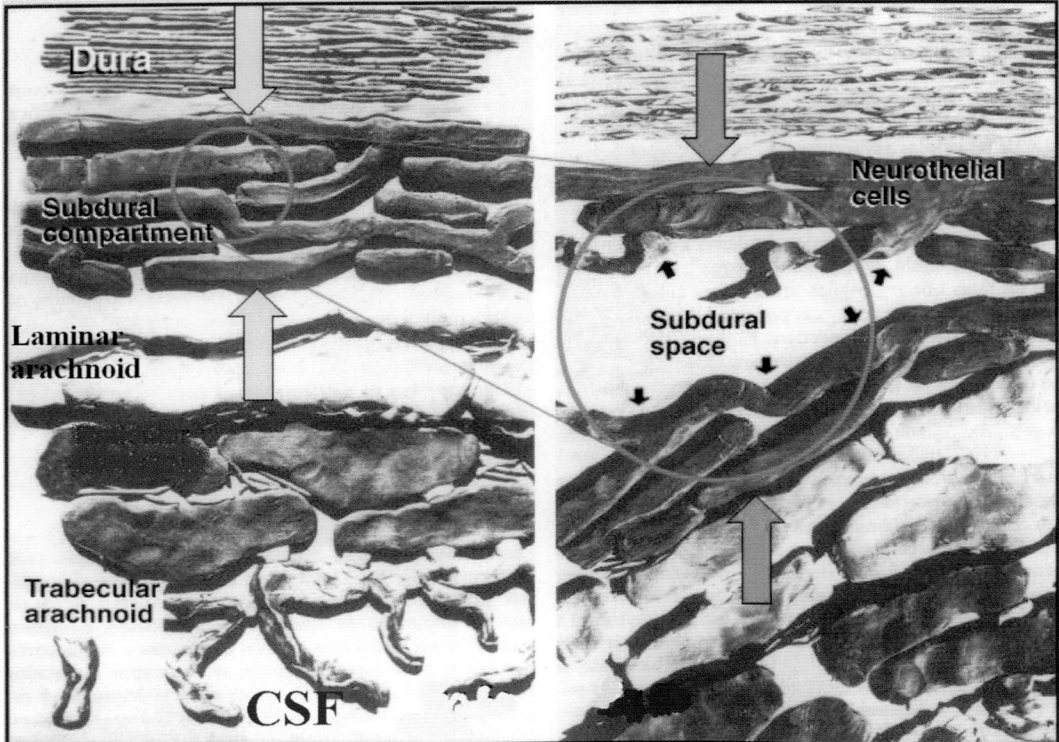

(a)

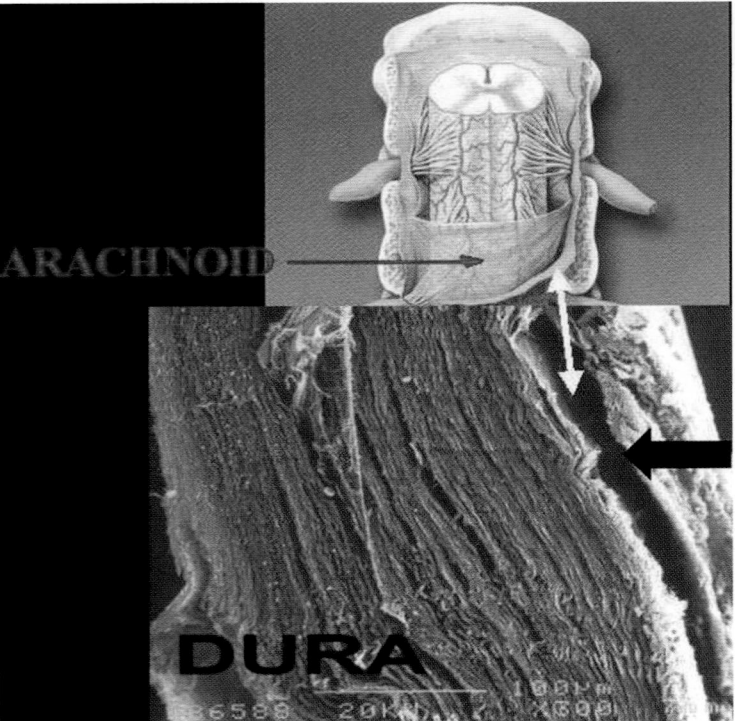

(b)

● **Fig. 5.16** (a) Two illustrations depicting the anatomy of the dura–arachnoid region, with an intact subdural compartment, at the dura–arachnoid interface, on the left, between the yellow arrows. On the right, the compartment has been disrupted, between the green arrows, creating a subdural space. (b) The upper illustration depicts the tearing away of the thick dura (yellow) from the filmy arachnoid, to create a subdural space, which is clearly seen in the lower electron microscope image (black arrow). (Both a and b are based on illustrations kindly supplied by Professor M. A. Reina, Madrid, Spain.)

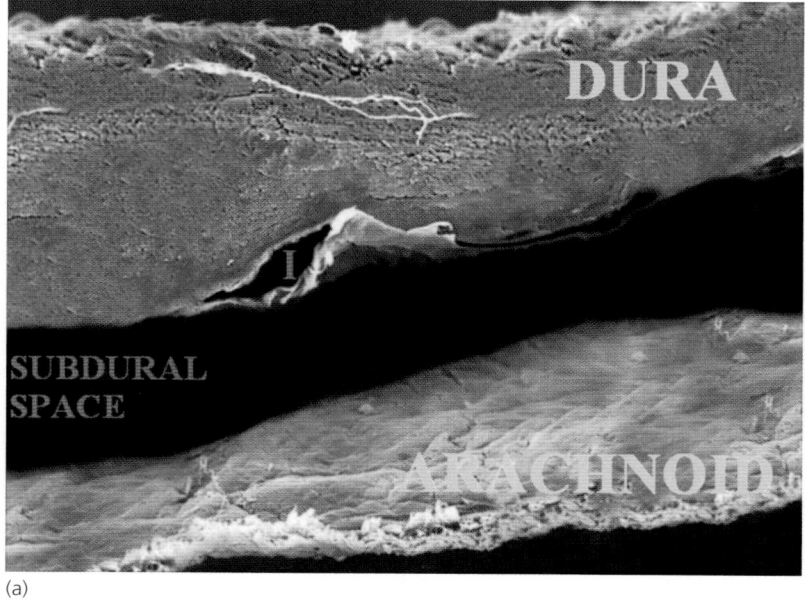

(a)

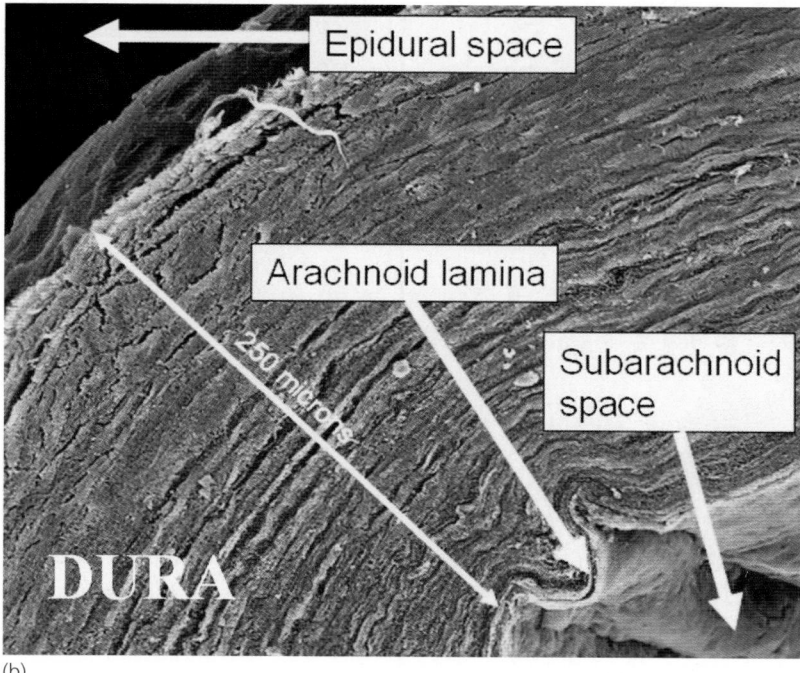

(b)

Fig. 5.17 (a) Scanning electron microscopy (SEM) image showing a subdural space between the dura and arachnoid. The intradural space (I) lies parallel to the subdural space, within the innermost layers of the dura. (b) An SEM image of the meninges showing the concentric rings formed by the dural laminae. Original magnification ×300.

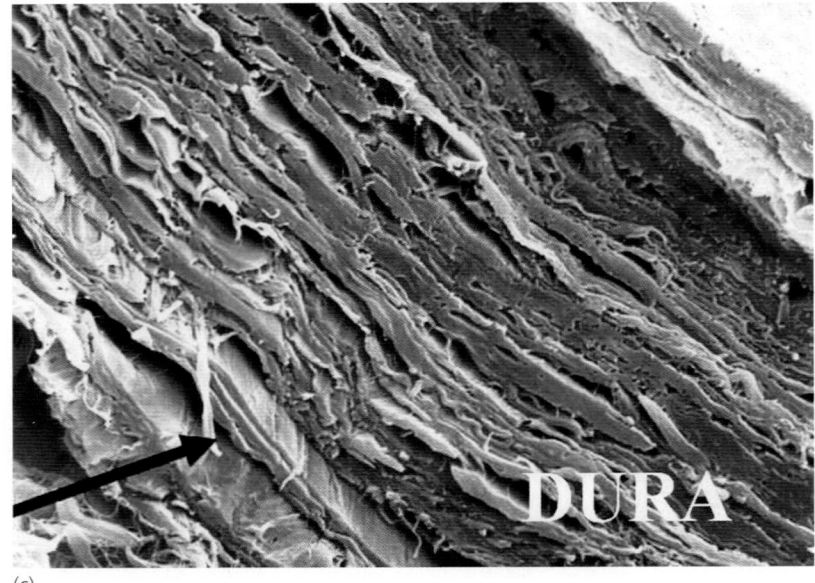

(c)

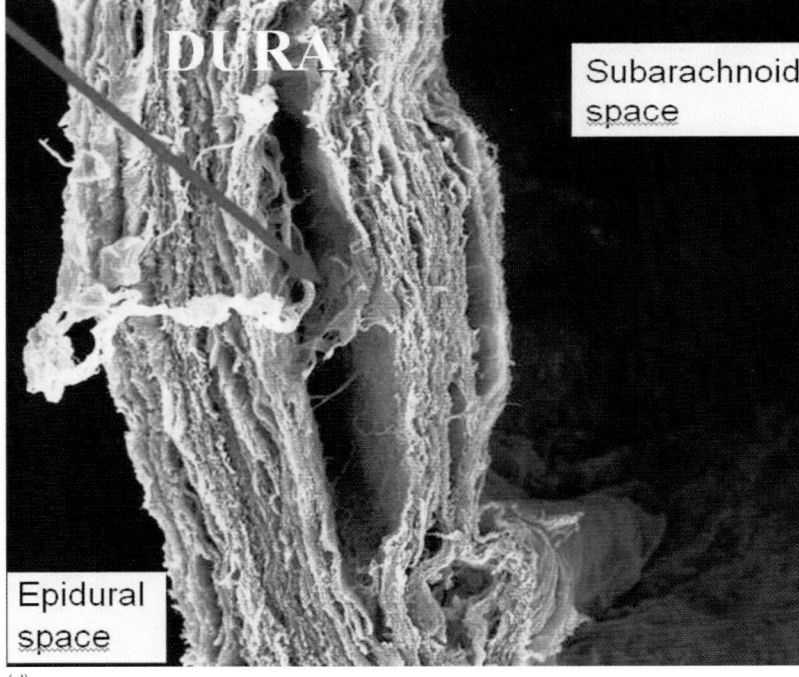

(d)

● **Fig. 5.17** (Continued) (c) An SEM view of concentric dural laminae and an enclosed artefactual intradural space (arrowed). Original magnification ×300. (d) An SEM view of dural laminae and an enclosed artefactual intradural space (arrowed). Original magnification ×300.

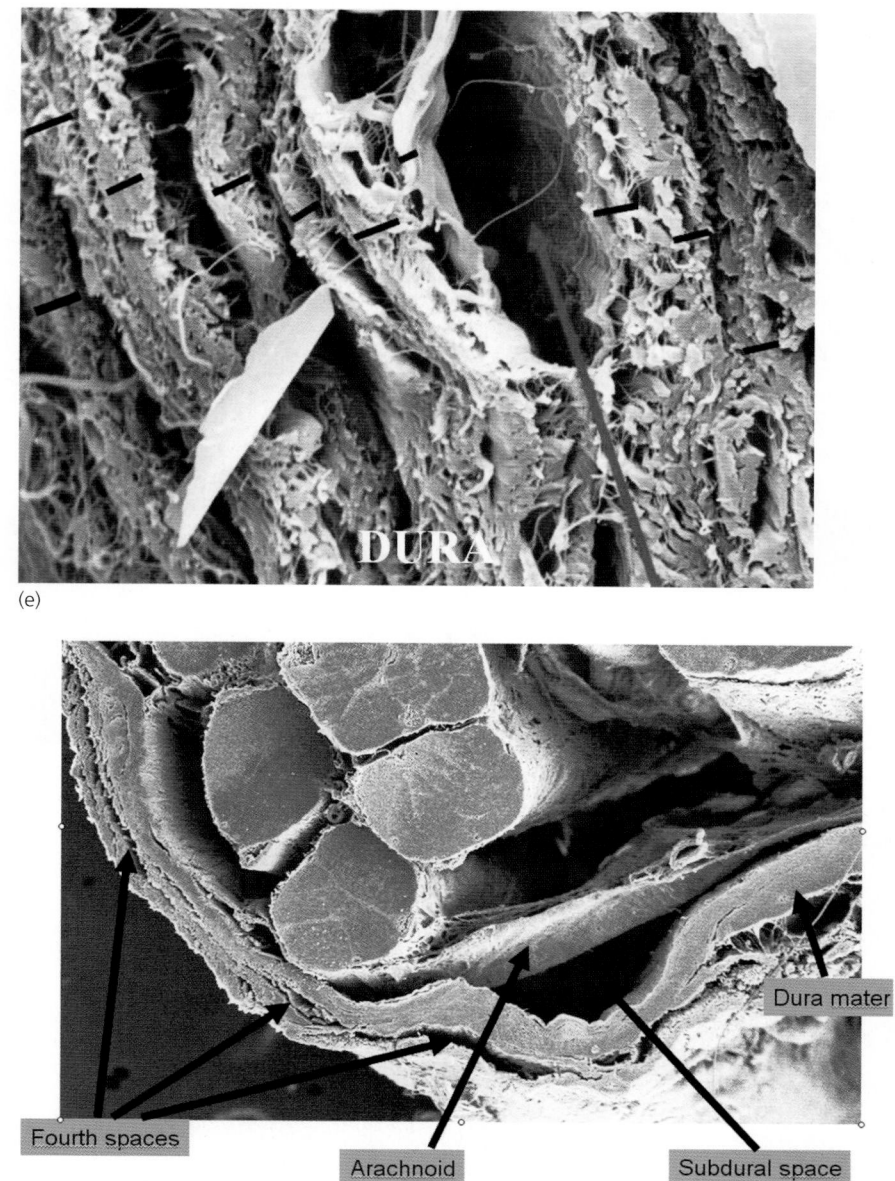

(e)

(f)

Fig. 5.17 (Continued) (e) Enhanced SEM image of individual dural laminae (black lines), surrounding an artefactual intradural space (arrowed). Original magnification ×2000. (f) An SEM image of the lumbar dural sac, with the nerve roots of the cauda equina above, enveloped in the arachnoid mater, and the presence of both intradural and subdural spaces. Original magnification ×25.

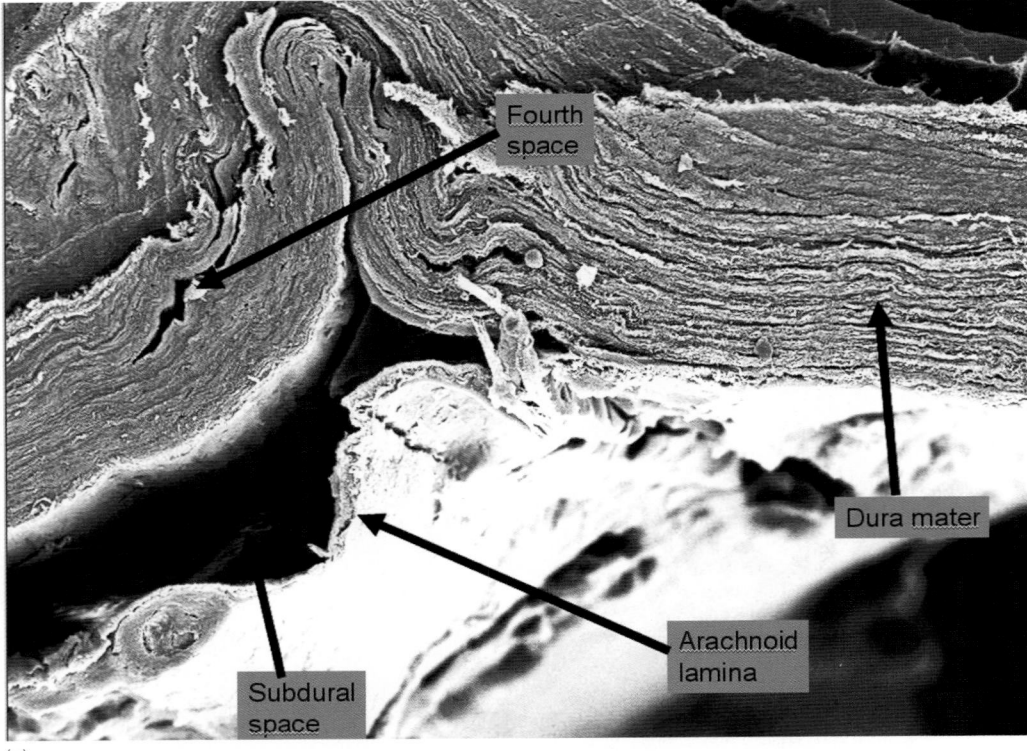

(g)

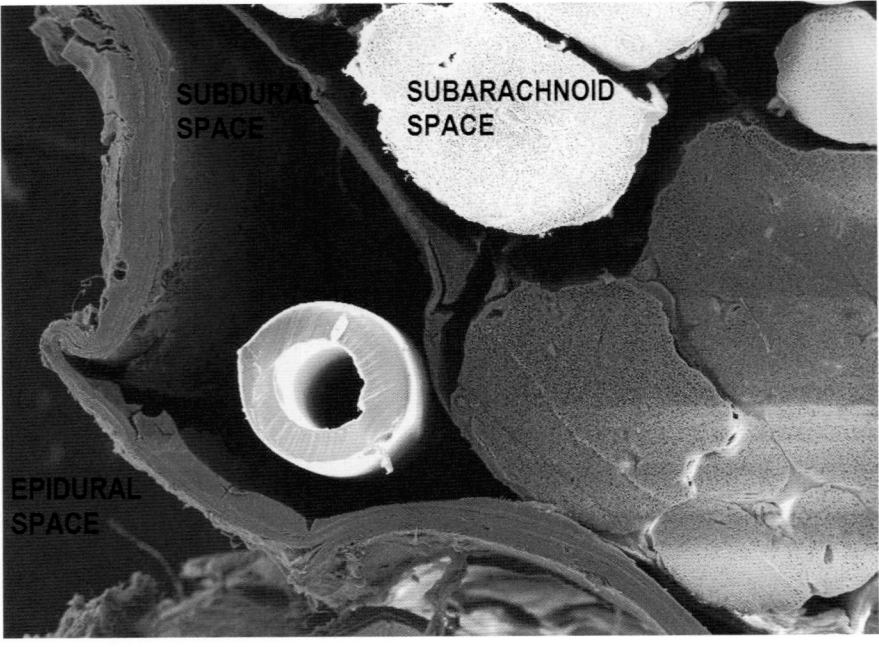

(h)

Fig. 5.17 (Continued) (g) An SEM image of lumbar meninges showing an intradural (or fourth) space and a subdural space. Original magnification ×25. (h) An SEM image revealing the presence of an epidural catheter within a lumbar subdural space. The nerve roots of the cauda equina lie above and to the right. Original magnification ×25.

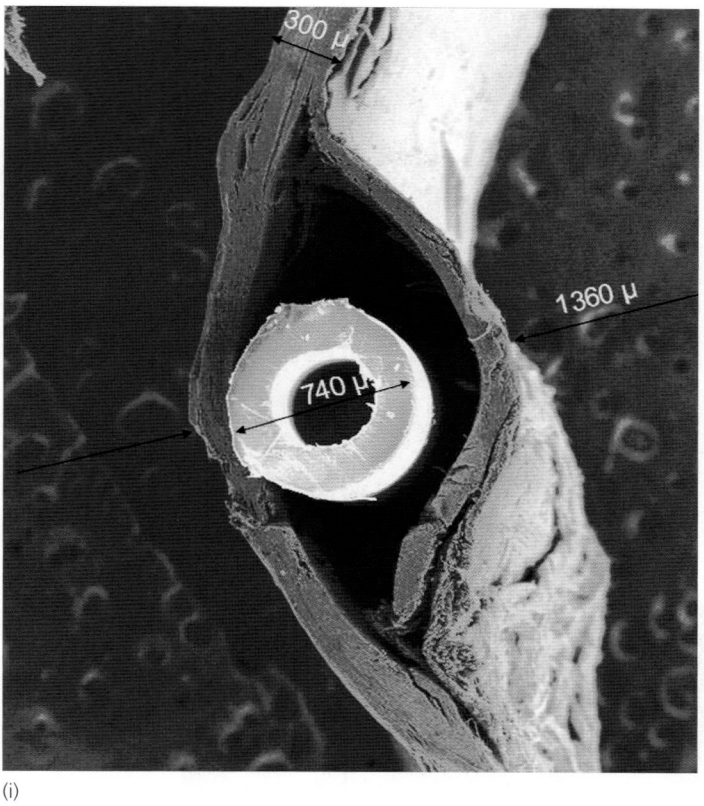

(i)

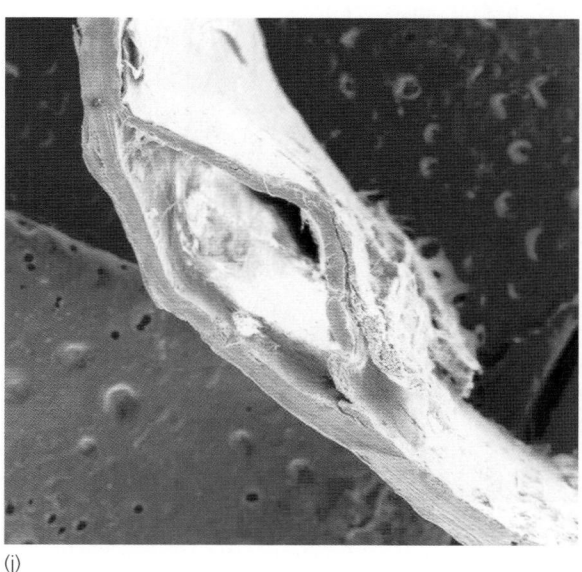

(j)

Fig. 5.17 (Continued) (i) An SEM image of an epidural catheter within the substance of the dura, or 'intradural', showing a dural thickness of 300 µm and a combined width of dura and catheter of 1360 µm. Original magnification ×25. (j) An SEM image (same specimen as in e) showing the cavity left behind within the dura following removal of an intradural catheter. Original magnification ×20.

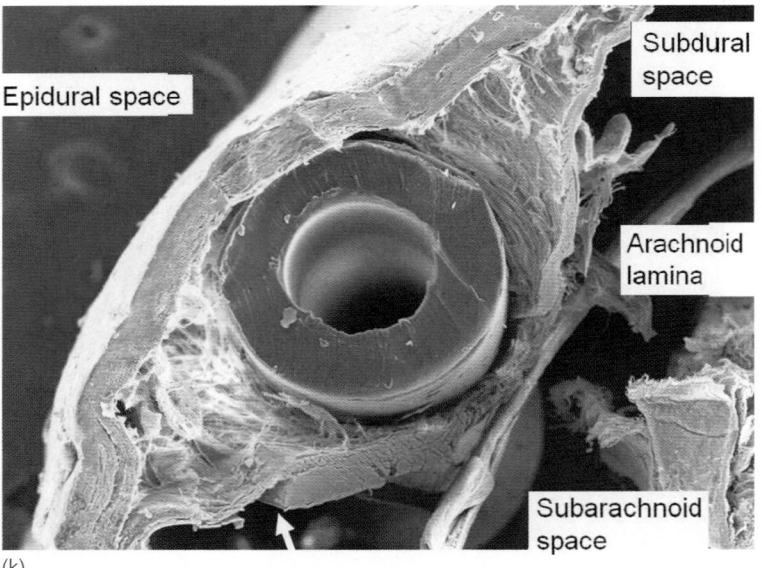

Epidural space

Subdural space

Arachnoid lamina

Subarachnoid space

(k)

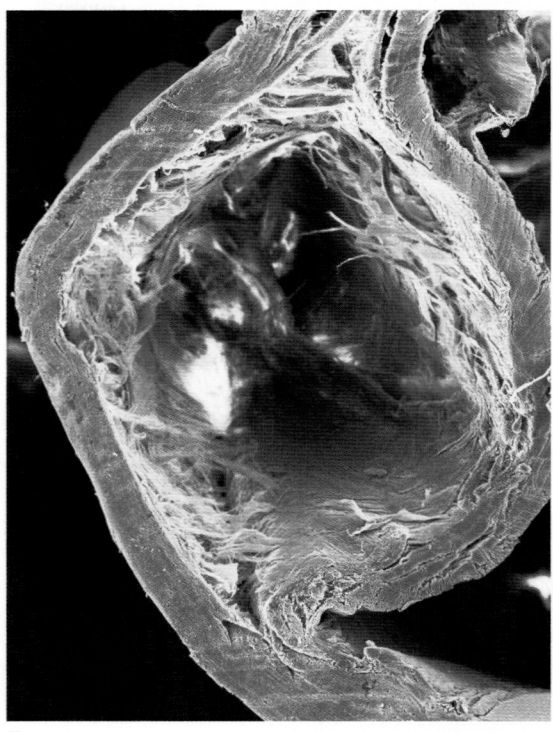

(l)

Fig. 5.17 (Continued) (k) An SEM image showing an epidural catheter migrating from an intradural space to the subarachnoid space, the arrow indicates an area of dural breakage. Original magnification ×40. (l) An SEM image (same specimen as in k) showing the cavity left behind within the dura following removal of an intradural catheter. Original magnification ×75. (All the SEM images are based on illustrations kindly supplied by Professor M. A. Reina, Madrid, Spain.)

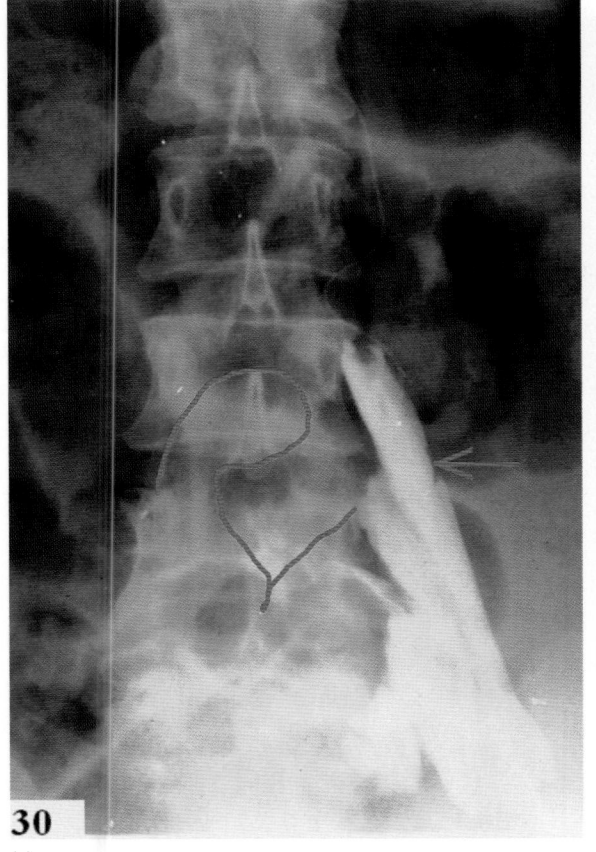

(a)

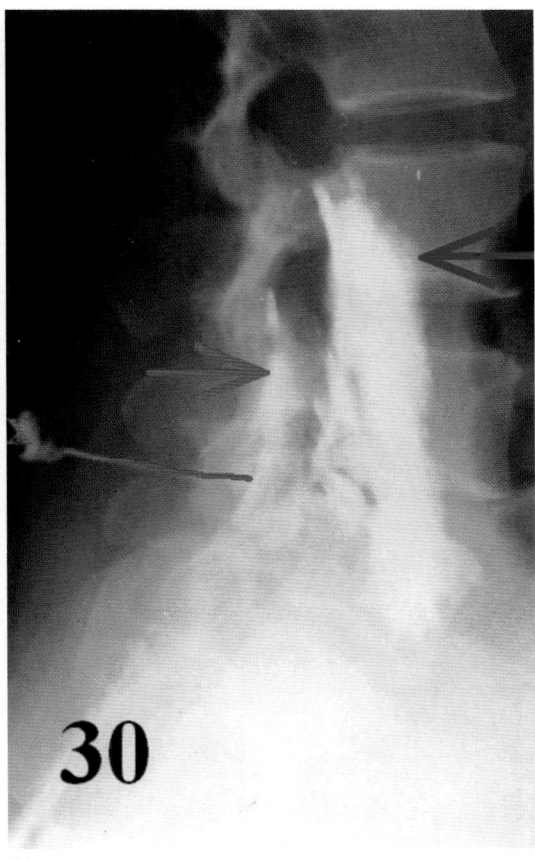

(b)

● **Fig. 6.2** (a) Anteroposterior (AP) epidurogram following catheter escape, with contrast outlining the tendinous insertion of the left psoas muscle (arrowed). For clarity only the distal portion of the catheter is highlighted. It proceeds towards and exits through the left L4–5 intervertebral foramen. (b) Lateral epidurogram following catheter escape, with contrast collecting behind the left psoas muscle (blue arrow). Following catheter withdrawal by 2 cm, further contrast injection enters the posterior epidural space (red arrow), with some extravasation to the skin (X).

entering the posterior epidural space (arrowed). Contrast is also seen flowing retrogradely to the skin insertion site (indicated by X), reflecting an increased pressure in the epidural space.

CASE HISTORY 6.3:
FAILED BLOCK

A total dose of 42 mL lidocaine 2% was injected over a 2-h period in a patient in labour through an epidural catheter, inserted at L1–2, with an intended 5 cm in the epidural space. This only resulted in sensory block of the right Ll and L2 dermatomes.

Epidurogram findings: transforaminal catheter escape

In the AP radiograph (Fig. 6.3) there is a mild degree of thoracolumbar scoliosis with the catheter tip

slightly to the right of the midline. The contrast is seen collecting anterior to the right psoas (arrowed), and the path of the catheter tip out through the right L1–2 intervertebral foramen is evident. Throughout this work, there appears to be an association between scoliosis and catheter escape, with the catheters tending to be (but not invariably) directed towards the inside of the thoracolumbar curve.

CASE HISTORY 6.4:
FAILED INITIAL BLOCK, SECOND CATHETER ADDED

The patient was 42 years old, and in her first labour. She gave a history of congenital right leg-shortening (5 cm) and moderate scoliosis. No analgesia resulted from her initial block at L3–4, with 5 cm of catheter being inserted

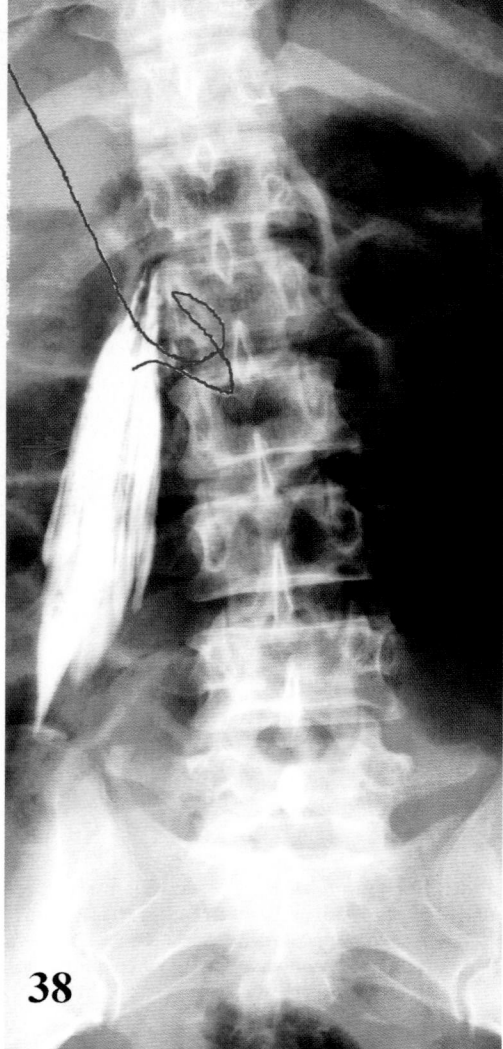

38

● **Fig. 6.3** Anteroposterior (AP) radiograph showing moderate scoliosis with the epidural catheter tip escaping through the right L1–2 intervertebral foramen and contrast highlighting the psoas muscle (arrowed).

into the epidural space. Withdrawal of the catheter by 1 cm, and an additional dose of local anaesthetic, had no effect. The catheter was left *in situ*, while another catheter was inserted successfully at L2–3.

Epidurogram findings: transforaminal escape/typical epidurogram
There was a moderate degree of thoracic scoliosis, with the primary curve to the right, and mild rotation of the lumbar vertebrae (Fig. 6.4). Both epidural catheters had been inserted just to the left of the midline. Under fluoroscopic control, contrast injection through the

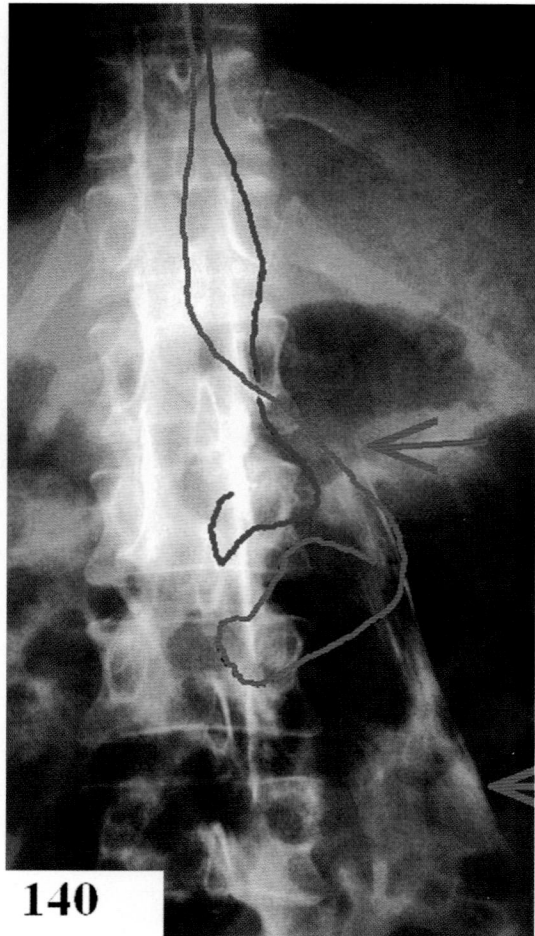

140

● **Fig. 6.4** Anteroposterior (AP) radiograph showing lower (red) catheter emerging through left L2–3 intervertebral foramen and contrast outlining the lateral border of the left psoas muscle (arrowed). Injection through the upper (blue) catheter results in epidural contrast spread between T10 and L4.

initial (red) catheter met with some resistance, and only 2 mL could be injected. The catheter was seen to exit the left L2–3 intervertebral foramen and proceed for some distance anterior to the psoas. The small volume of contrast flowed rapidly to outline the lateral border of the psoas (arrowed, Fig. 6.4). Injection through the upper (blue) catheter produced a fairly typical, but restricted, bilateral contrast spread from T10 to L4.

6.1.2 Partial catheter escape

As will be noted in Case Histories 6.5 and 6.6, the proportion of contrast flowing into the epidural space, rather than escaping through a foramen, seemed to depend on the positioning of the catheter tip, the location of the eyes, and probably the injection pressure used.[4]

CASE HISTORY 6.5:
PARTIALLY INADEQUATE EPIDURAL BLOCK

A labouring patient of small stature (height 150 cm, pre-pregnant weight 51 kg) was unusual in view of the extremely shallow depth of her epidural space and presumed bilateral catheter escapes. Initially, the L3–4 epidural space was located at a depth of only 2.5 cm and a catheter inserted to leave 3.5 cm in the space. A dose of 10 mL bupivacaine 0.375% produced only numbness of the left thigh (L2–3), which could not be improved by withdrawing the catheter by 1 cm and administering a further dose. The catheter was removed and another inserted 2.5 cm into the epidural space at L2–3 (depth of the epidural space now 2.75 cm). A repeat dose of local anaesthetic produced good pain relief for labour with a T9 sensory level, but a heavy right leg (Bromage 2) and inadequate sensory block for forceps delivery.

Epidurogram findings: partial transforaminal escape
The AP epidurogram (Fig. 6.5a) reveals the catheter tip to be emerging through the right L2–3 intervertebral foramen with the characteristic anterior psoas highlighting (red arrow), together with limited and patchy

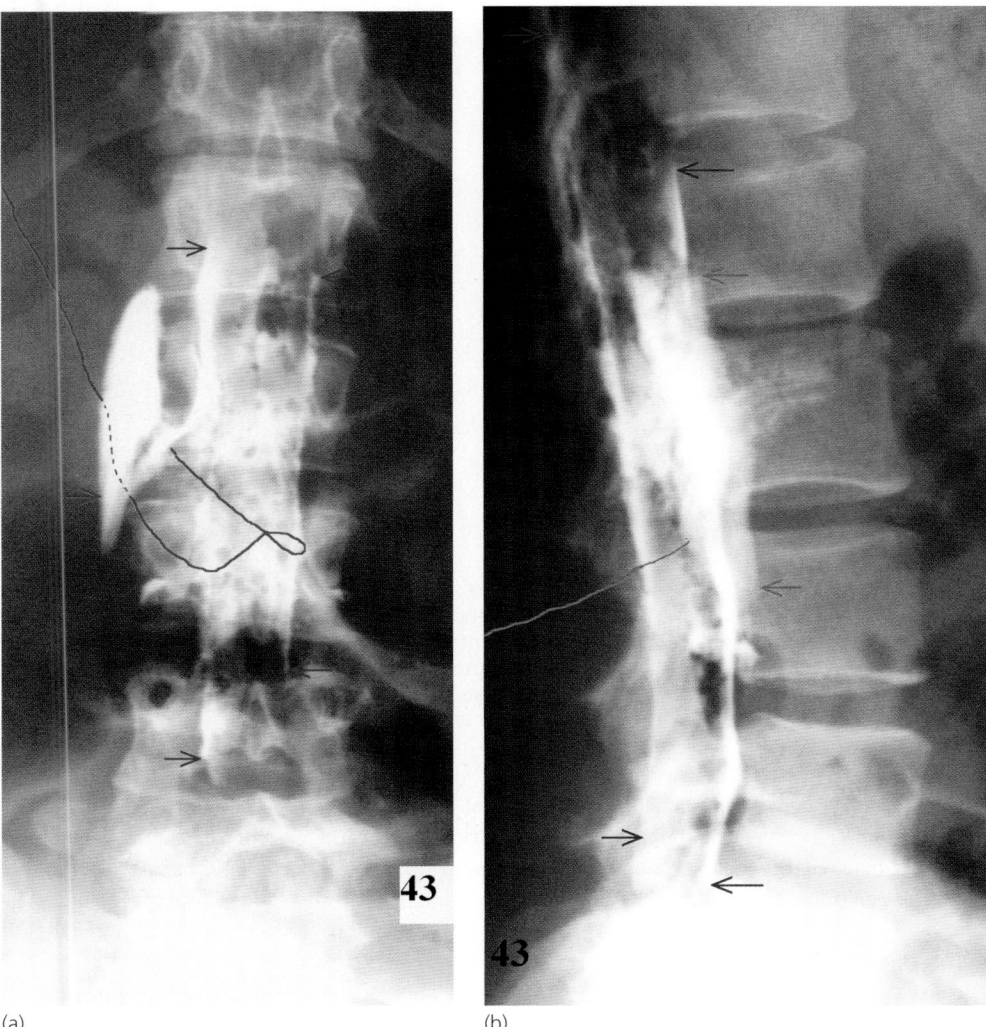

(a)   (b)

● **Fig. 6.5** (a) Anteroposterior (AP) radiograph showing the epidural catheter emerging through the right L2–3 intervertebral foramen, with contrast highlighting the right psoas muscle (red arrow). Limited epidural spread is evident between L1 and L4 bilaterally (blue arrows). (b) Lateral radiograph. The epidural catheter is seen to enter the mass of psoas contrast (red arrows), which overlies the limited spread of epidural contrast (blue arrows).

epidural filling from L1 to L4 (blue arrows). The lateral view (Fig. 6.5b) shows the restricted epidural filling from Ll to S1, with the psoas collection (red arrows) overlying the L1–L3 vertebral bodies and the anterior and posterior epidural columns of contrast (blue arrows).

CASE HISTORY 6.6:
PARTIALLY INADEQUATE EPIDURAL BLOCK

A 34-year-old patient received an epidural block at L3–4 in labour. The 'closer-eye' catheter (Portex) had three lateral eyes at 2, 3 and 4 mm from a closed tip. It was inserted to leave a length of 4 cm in the epidural space. The block was totally right-sided, from T8 to L1, despite repeated doses of local anaesthetic and withdrawal of the catheter by 1 cm. Delivery occurred with minimal analgesia.

Epidurogram findings: partial transforaminal escape
On screening and contrast injection, the catheter could be seen emerging from the right L2–3 foramen and contrast initially highlighted the psoas muscle (Fig. 6.6). Ten seconds later, a narrow lateral column of epidural contrast appeared on the right. Over the next 20 s, both collections of contrast expanded, but the epidural column did not extend beyond L1–L4 (Fig. 6.6).

In summary, cases of partial epidural block with some degree of catheter escape may present as difficult clinical diagnostic problems, and epidurography may be the only means of resolution.[5] Because of the small volume of local anaesthetic that actually finds its way to the epidural space, the block will be restricted and often patchy, but the effects of any accompanying unilateral lumbar plexus block may confuse the situation. Depending on the volume and concentration of the escaping local anaesthetic and the path taken, lumbar plexus block may result in blockade of one or two of the adjacent L1, L2 or L3 dermatomes, with occasional lumbar sympathetic block or, rarely, moderate quadriceps weakness.

If a plexus block is present, cases of transforaminal escape without any epidural component can usually be diagnosed by simple clinical examination of the extent of the block, and epidurography is not required. On most occasions, however, no lumbar plexus block is detectable, and the block is a total failure.

An epidurogram revealing catheter escape may highlight a very shallow depth of the epidural space, such as 2.5 cm, as in Case History 6.4. Such a finding should be recorded and the patient notified in case of future need for epidural block.

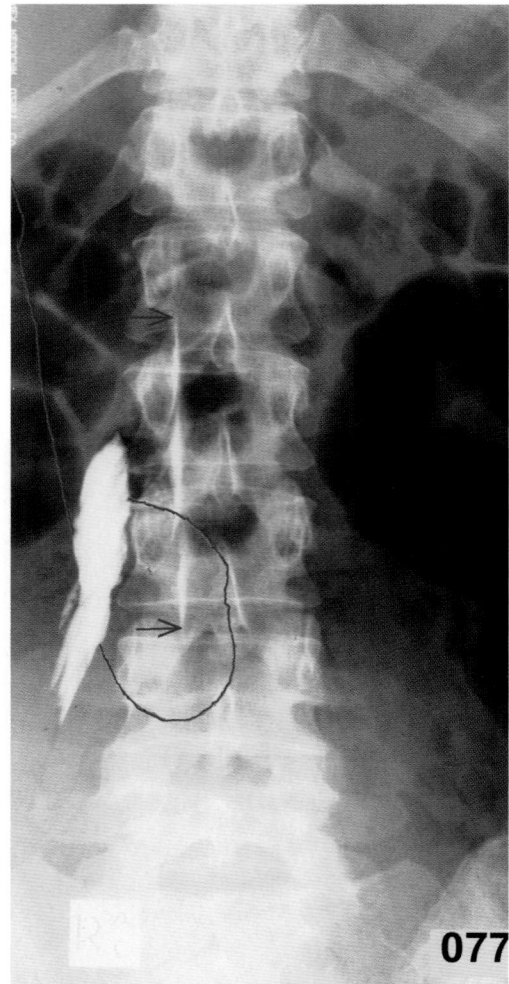

077

● **Fig. 6.6** Anteroposterior (AP) radiograph depicting the epidural catheter emerging through the right L2–3 intervertebral foramen with contrast highlighting the right psoas muscle. Limited epidural spread is evident between L1 and L4 (arrowed).

With regard to epidural catheter design, the development of an instance of partial transforaminal escape with a 'closer-eye' catheter is of interest, as it suggests that even with eyes positioned 1 mm apart, solutions may flow simultaneously into the epidural space and escape into the paravertebral space. It should also be noted that the passage of an epidural catheter through an intervertebral foramen was not associated with any unusual paraesthesiae, which might have been of diagnostic value. Catheter design and the propensity to escape is discussed in Chapter 9 (see section 9.5.2, p.127).

6.2 Paravertebral catheter placement

An unusual cause of epidural failure is occasionally seen when the epidural needle and catheter are inadvertently directed laterally and away from the epidural space towards the paravertebral region. Depending on the positioning of the catheter and the dose of local anaesthetic injected, a variable degree of unilateral paravertebral block may develop.

CASE HISTORY 6.7:
LIMITED UNILATERAL PARAVERTEBRAL BLOCK

Epidural catheter insertion at L2–3 was attempted on a 38-year-old obese (125 kg) patient undergoing gynaecological surgery. Although no distinctive loss of resistance was detected, a 4 cm length of a terminal-eye wire-reinforced catheter (Arrow International, Reading, PA, USA) was passed easily through the Tuohy needle. Twenty minutes after a dose of 20 mL lidocaine 2% a limited left-sided sensory block developed from T10 to L1. A further injection of 10 mL increased the extent of the blocked area, which was now from T9 to L2, with sensory loss only. General anaesthesia was instituted before surgery.

Epidurogram findings: left paravertebral contrast
On fluoroscopy, the radio-opaque epidural catheter can be seen to have been inserted in the midline at L1–2, but then to run laterally around the L2 vertebral body and come to rest, with the tip coiled up, in the left paravertebral gutter. The first 6 mL of contrast was seen to accumulate in the left paravertebral space between T10 and L2, and then spread medially as a dense but fragmented mass (AP view, Fig. 6.7a). Another 6 mL of contrast extended the flow vertically and medially to cross the midline. The lateral view (Fig. 6.7b) again reveals a dense and patchy mass of contrast in the paravertebral region between T10 and L2 spreading around the T10–L2 vertebral bodies and collecting anterior to them. This scattered radiographic pattern is quite different from the psoasgram following catheter escape. The more extensive unilateral sensory block after paravertebral block may allow the diagnosis to be made on clinical examination alone, but the differential diagnosis between a unilateral epidural block and an extensive paravertebral block may be difficult without epidurography.

6.3 Retrograde flow and extravasation of epidural solutions

Retrograde flow of contrast with extravasation into the muscles of the back or to the skin may produce some unusual and confusing images in AP radiographs, but the lateral views readily reveal the contrast to have escaped from the epidural space by retrograde flow (and sometimes exited the patient's body as well).

There are two possible mechanisms that may lead to retrograde flow, which we considered significant in 4% of our patients. First, and more commonly, the catheter has accidentally been partially or completely withdrawn from a correct position in the epidural space and comes to rest with one or more of its eyes outside the space, or even further out, in the erector spinae muscles. Escaping local anaesthetic, or later contrast, follows the path of least resistance and may exit along the track of the catheter before forming a collection under the skin-fixation covering the insertion site.

Second, extravasation back along the outside of a correctly sited epidural catheter may occur when excessive pressure builds up during injection into an epidural space that is restricted by a septum, adhesions or bony abnormality, and retrograde flow occurs. Several examples of this are seen as incidental findings in the epidurograms following unilateral block, as shown in Chapter 7 (see Fig. 7.3a–c, pp.86–87).

Extravasation of epidural local anaesthetic solutions to the skin may loosen the fixation being used and allow for the catheter to be expelled prematurely.[6] We have seen many examples of this when patients that have repeated blocks for successive childbirth report that their catheters 'always fall out early'.

An unusual case of retrograde flow with extravasation, but without any obvious major anatomical defect is described in Case History 6.8.

CASE HISTORY 6.8:
RETROGRADE FLOW OF CONTRAST

Epidural block at L3–4 in a primiparous labour appeared to be uneventful, with 4 cm of catheter being inserted into the epidural space; however, it only resulted in a very patchy block, despite repeated doses of local anaesthetic. The skin-fixation over the epidural puncture site was removed before catheter reinsertion at L2–3, and found to be saturated with leaking local anaesthetic solution. The first catheter was left *in situ*, and a second block

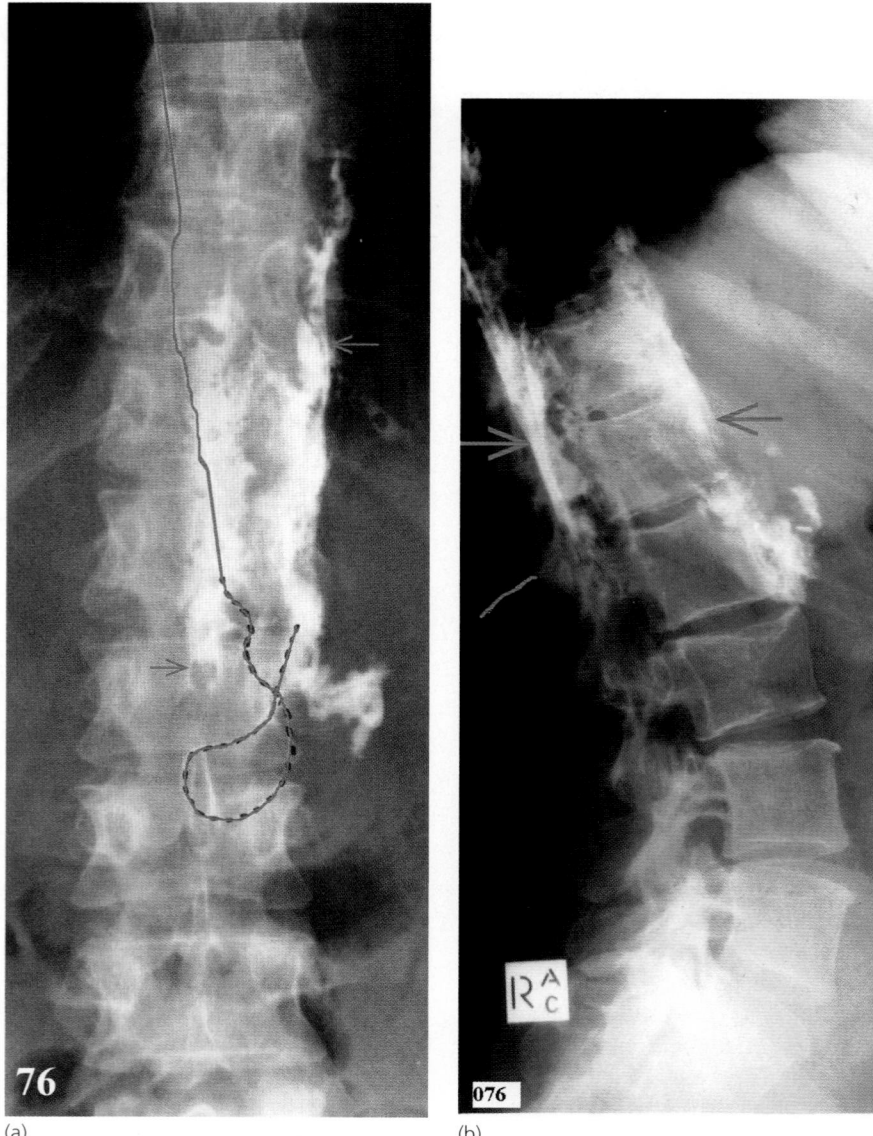

(a)   (b)

● **Fig. 6.7** (a) Anteroposterior (AP) radiograph, with epidural catheter entering a left paravertebral mass of contrast, which has spread anteriorly to the midline (between the arrows) from T10 to L2. (b) Lateral radiograph showing a collection of paravertebral contrast that has spread anteriorly (between the arrows) from T10 to L2.

inserted without difficulty. This proved to be entirely satisfactory.

Epidurogram findings: 1. left paravertebral contrast; 2. slightly restricted epidural contrast pattern

Fluoroscopy the following day revealed a mild thoracolumbar scoliosis (primary curve convex to the right), with both catheter tips appearing to be placed

in the midline. Contrast injected into the lower epidural catheter (Fig. 6.8a, coloured red) at L3 produced only a small and very faint localized collection in the epidural space, before it leaked retrogradely around the catheter producing two distinct dense irregular masses of contrast external to the vertebral column (AP view, Fig. 6.8a, red arrows). Injection through the upper (blue) catheter at L2 now resulted in a fairly normal spread of contrast, but with restricted vertical spread (Fig. 6.8b).

● **Fig. 7.2** (a) Anteroposterior (AP) radiograph showing a midline fissure (arrowed) within the body of contrast, indicating a dorsal midline septum. The mass of contrast is narrow and tapers off at T10 and there is little foraminal escape of contrast, both of which are features that suggest the contrast lies predominantly at the back of the epidural space. (b) Lateral radiograph confirming the predominant posterior distribution of the contrast, with a large central filling defect (arrowed), representing a probable transverse extension of a midline septum. A small volume of contrast surrounds the catheter within the erector spinae muscles.

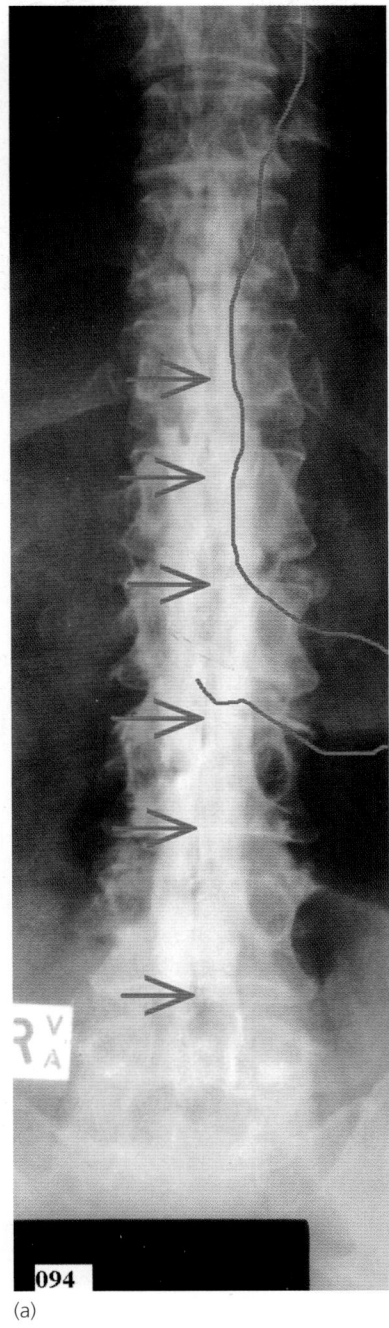

(a)

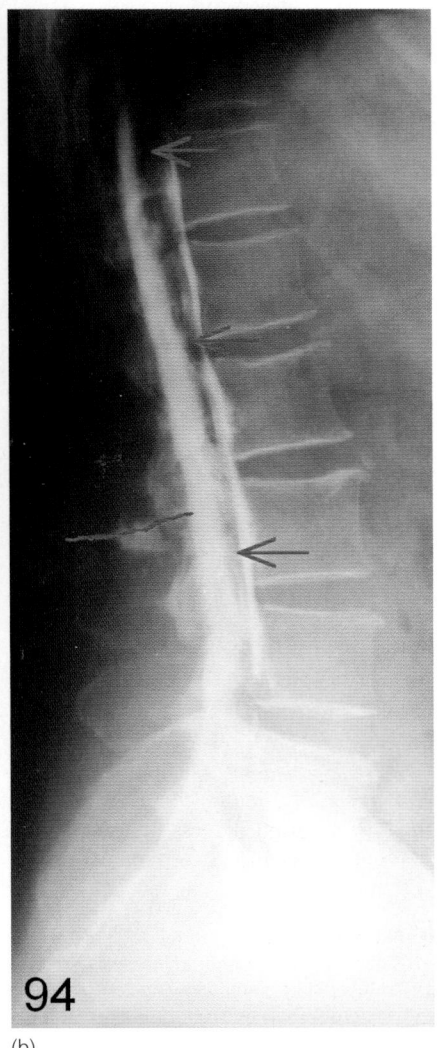

(b)

7.5.1 The midline septum

UNILATERAL BLOCK

Two epidural catheters (three lateral eyes; Portex) were required for effective analgesia in a patient during her first labour. The first catheter had been inserted at L2–3, with 3 cm entering the epidural space. Despite 20 mL bupivacaine 0.375% and catheter withdrawal by 1 cm, the block remained totally unilateral on the left. A second catheter was then inserted at L1–2, to a similar depth, and increments of bupivacaine injected. It was not until a further 15 mL had been given over 20 min, that satisfactory bilateral block developed.

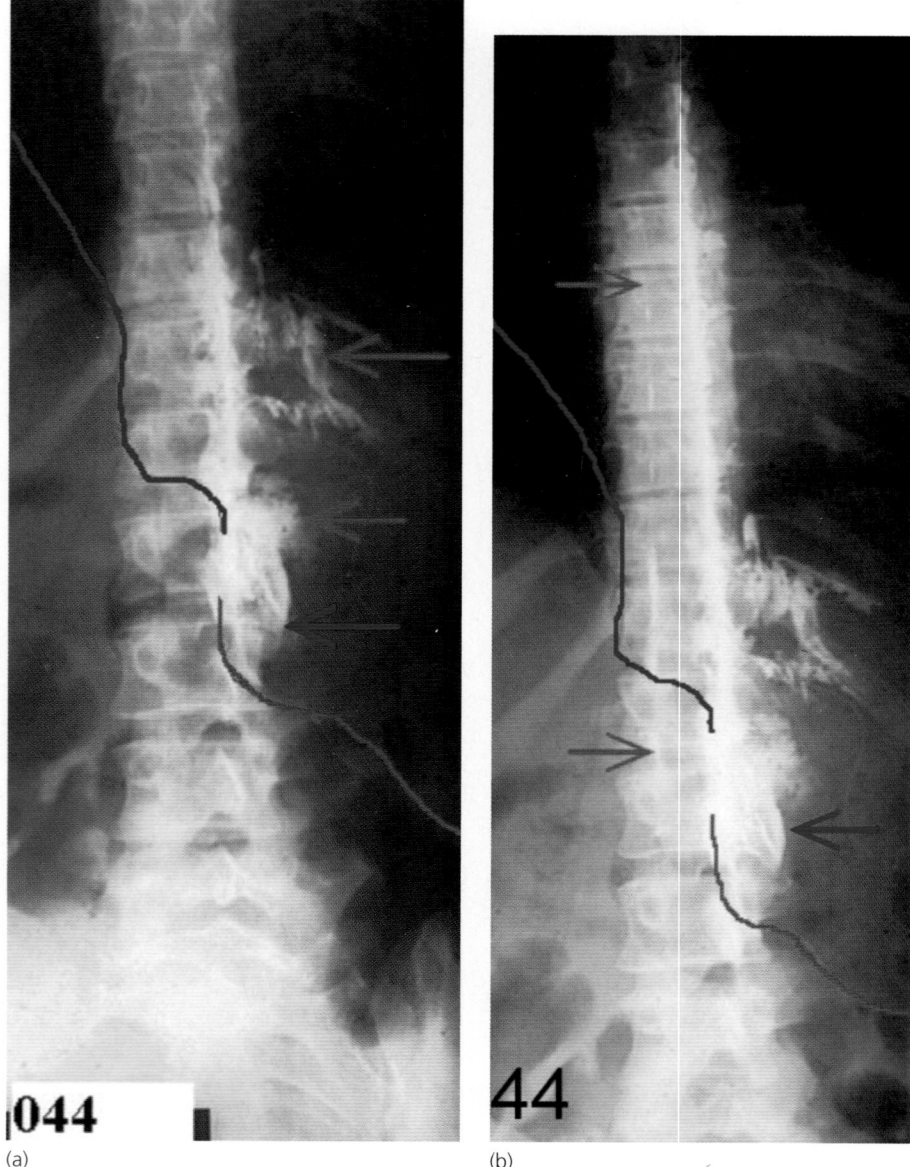

(a) (b)

● **Fig. 7.3** (a) Anteroposterior (AP) epidurogram following contrast injection through the lower (red) catheter. Contrast is totally left-sided, with profuse foraminal spill (red arrows) and retrograde flow to the erector spinae muscles and skin (blue arrow). (b) An AP epidurogram following contrast injection through the upper (blue) catheter. Initially, the contrast remains left-sided, with increasing spill and retrograde flow (blue arrow). Later, contrast appears on the right as an attenuated and fragmented lateral column from T8 to L2 (red arrows).

Epidurogram findings: **dorsal midline septum**

The first AP epidurogram (Fig. 7.3a) reveals a mild degree of thoracolumbar scoliosis, with slight rotation of the vertebral bodies to the left. On screening, the two epidural catheter tips were found to be positioned almost adjacent to one another, well to the left of the midline at L2. The first 10 mL of contrast given through the lower

(red) catheter produced only a left-sided channelling with profuse spill of contrast through the T11–L2 intervertebral foramina (red arrows). The L1–2 spill is partially obscured by retrograde flow of contrast to the skin and paravertebral muscles (blue arrow).

The first 4 mL through the upper (blue) catheter was also left-sided, with the initial column of contrast

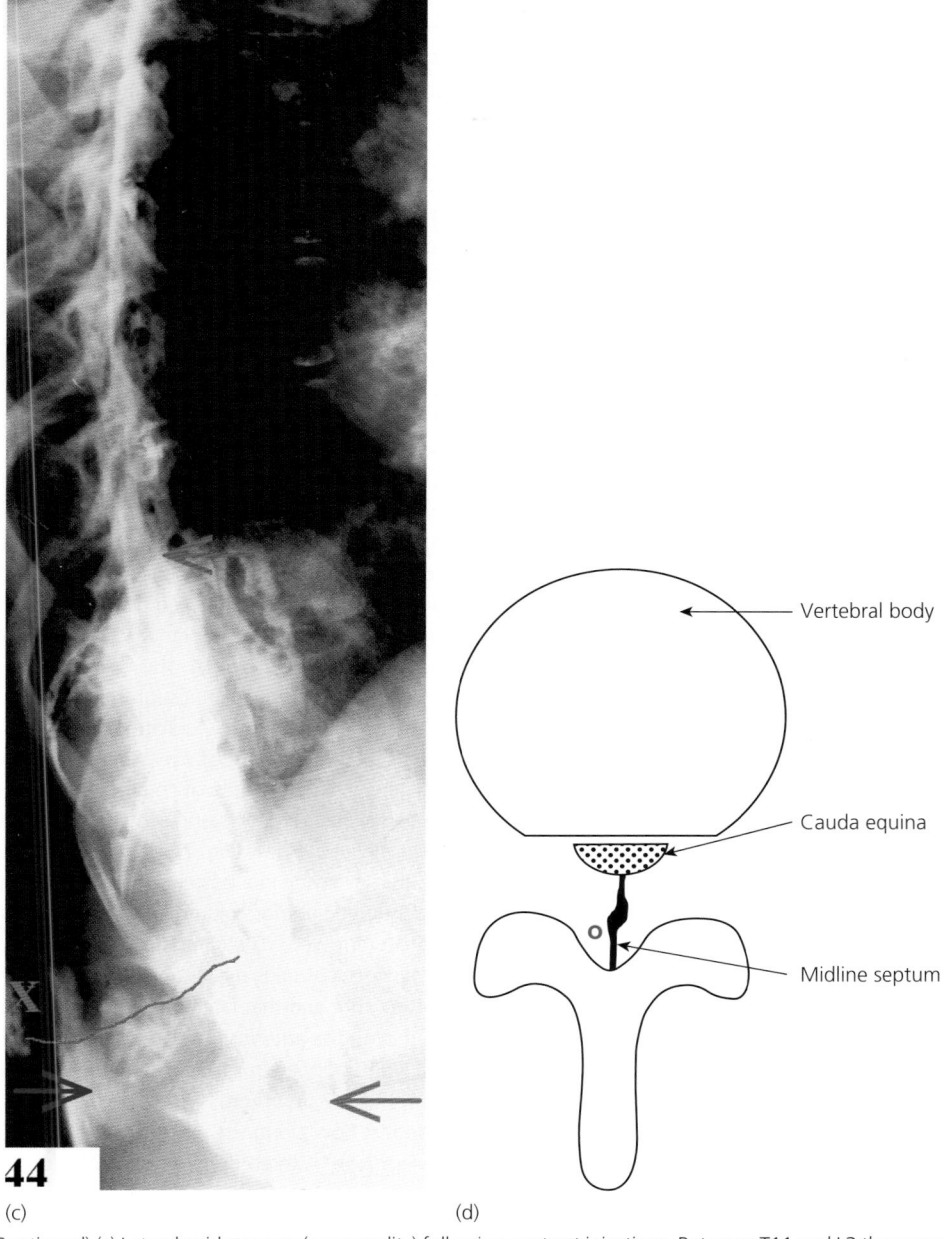

Vertebral body

Cauda equina

Midline septum

44

(c)   (d)

● **Fig. 7.3** (Continued) (c) Lateral epidurogram (poor quality) following contrast injections. Between T11 and L3 there appears to be uniform spread of contrast across the epidural space (red arrows), with no evidence of a transverse septum. There is a high posterior contrast column up to T5. Retrograde flow of contrast is seen around the lower (red) catheter to the erector spinae muscles (blue arrow), and this partly obscures the mass of epidural contrast. Contrast leakage to the skin is evident (X). The upper catheter is not visible. (d) Diagram of septal anatomy and presumed position of the catheter tip (O), on the left side of the epidural space, in the same patient.

thickening, and showing increasing foraminal spill and retrograde flow (Fig. 7.3b). After a further 2 mL, contrast finally appeared on the right, as a very attenuated lateral column from T8–L2 (red arrows). On screening, this restricted right-sided filling commenced at L2 and then ran rostrally. This contralateral spread presumably flowed around the caudal end of the septum.

The lateral view (Fig. 7.3c) reveals the spread of contrast to be fairly uniform across the lumbar epidural space, suggesting the presence of a true midline septum

87

without lateral extensions, as shown in Fig. 7.3d, with the catheter position as indicated (O). The pressure generated in the left side of the epidural space during contrast injection appears to have been quite high in view of the copious volumes of contrast escaping through the foramina and even back along the outside of the catheter to the erector spinae muscles (Fig. 7.3c, blue arrow) and the skin (X).

In this case the first catheter had little or no function, but in some others it was found to be beneficial to have two catheters present, especially if they were positioned on either side of a septum, when they could be used simultaneously if required to produce adequate block.

CASE HISTORY 7.2:
PREDOMINANTLY UNILATERAL BLOCK

A 29-year-old patient developed a mainly left-sided block with persistent right lower abdominal pain throughout labour, following insertion of a terminal eye catheter (Portex) to a depth of 4 cm in the epidural space at L2–3. A further dose of 30 mL bupivacaine 0.375%, over 2 h, did not improve the quality or extent of the block.

Epidurogram findings: dorsal midline septum
Anteroposterior fluoroscopic screening (Fig. 7.4a) revealed the catheter tip to be in the midline at L2, with an extensive narrow left-sided column of contrast from T5 to L5 (Fig. 7.4a), filling at the same time as limited midline spread at T11–T12. After 20 s, a restricted and attenuated right-sided column of contrast developed from T11–L3. The AP radiograph (Fig. 7.4a) shows the predominantly left-sided contrast (arrowed), and the presence of bilateral foraminal spill at all levels where contrast is present. A midline septum is the most likely cause of this picture of contrast maldistribution. This is confirmed by the lateral view (Fig. 7.4b), which shows uniform spread of contrast across the epidural space from T12 to L5 (arrowed). Above this level, the posterior column of contrast is prominent up to T5, but a small volume of contrast again spreads across the epidural space.

7.5.2 Combined midline and transverse septum

In Case Histories 7.3 and 7.4, a midline septum is also present, but with the addition of lateral extensions, which form a transverse septum across the epidural space.

CASE HISTORY 7.3:
UNILATERAL BLOCK

A patient scheduled for elective caesarean section underwent uncomplicated epidural catheter insertion at L3–4, but following an incremental injection of 25 mL lidocaine 2% with adrenaline, the block remained totally left-sided, up to T4. The catheter was removed and another inserted at L2–3. Following a further 14 mL of local anaesthetic, patchy right-sided block developed. Despite the imperfect block, the patient was keen to remain awake for surgery and was comfortable, except for some moderately severe central abdominal pain during uterine manipulation.

Epidurogram findings: midline septum with lateral extensions
The AP epidurogram (Fig. 7.5a) reveals the tip of the catheter to be at L2–3, to the left of the midline, with almost totally left-sided spread of contrast and abundant foraminal spill from L1–L5. There is an almost straight line separating the unblocked right side from the left, although a very small volume of contrast can be detected 'leaking' to the right at L4. This was the only case in this work with a suspected septum where the contrast remained almost entirely unilateral. In view of the eventual development of a reasonable bilateral block for surgery, a larger volume of contrast than the 13 mL used may well have shown significant bilateral spread.

In the lateral view (Fig. 7.5b) the contrast is seen to collect mostly in a posterior column, with a fairly attenuated anterior column, separated by a large filling defect (arrowed). The combined radiographs suggest that a midline septum is preventing contrast flowing from left to right and that lateral extensions of the septum are impeding the anterior flow of contrast from a catheter tip (O) positioned in the left posterior dorsolateral space (Fig. 7.5c). There is evidence of faint retrograde contrast flow along the outside of the catheter at L2–3 in Fig. 7.5b. A three-dimensional model of the unilateral contrast spread is provided in Fig. 7.5d.

CASE HISTORY 7.4:
RECURRING UNILATERAL BLOCK

Prior to elective caesarean section, a patient reported that her previous epidural block in labour had remained largely right-sided, with only limited pain relief on the left side. A similar situation developed on this occasion following puncture at L2–3, with 6 cm of a three lateral eye catheter (Portex) in the epidural space. The right side was blocked to T10 but the left side only below

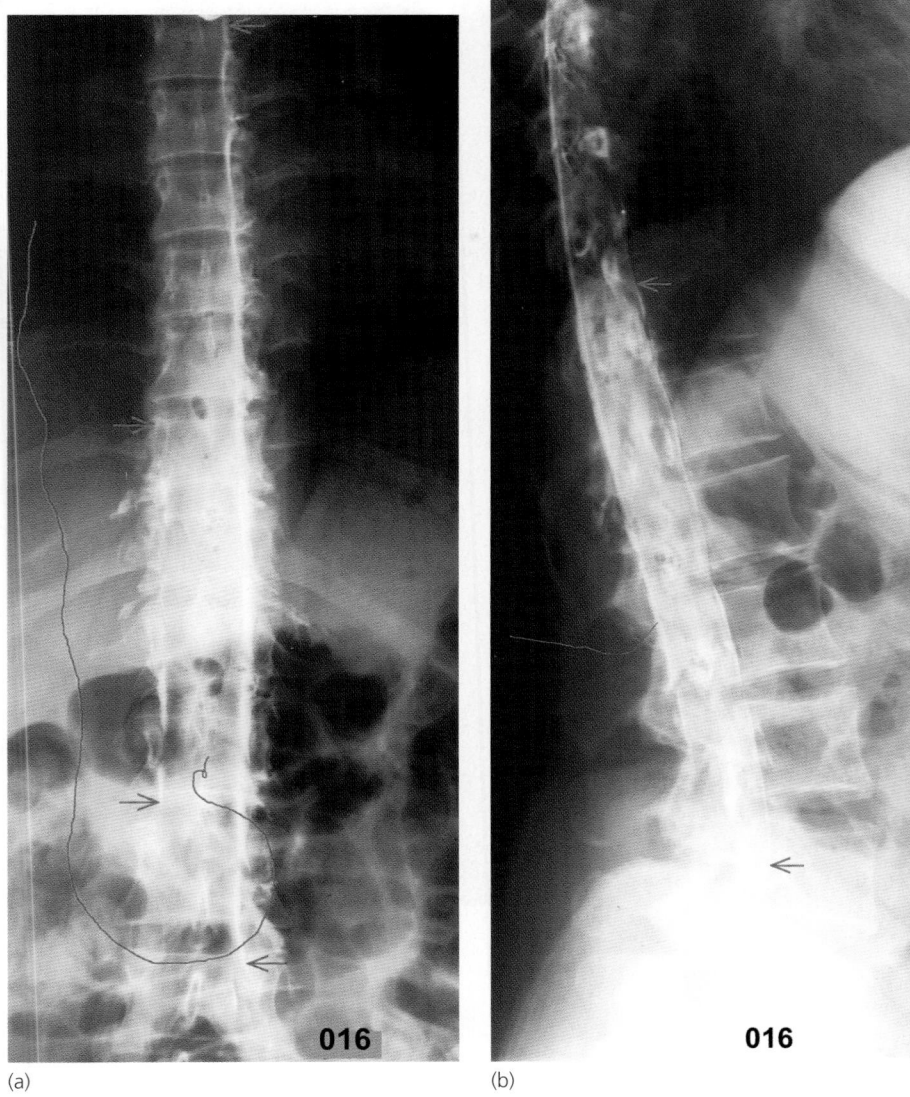

(a)   (b)

Fig. 7.4 (a) Anteroposterior (AP) epidurogram showing predominantly left-sided spread of contrast (T5 to L5, arrowed) from a centrally placed catheter tip, almost certainly caused by a midline septum. The attenuated right-sided contrast only extends from T11 to L3. (b) Lateral epidurogram following unilateral block, with uniform spread of contrast across the lumbar epidural space (from T12 to L5, arrowed), suggesting a midline septum with no lateral extensions.

L4 following an injection of 16 mL bupivacaine 0.5%. Withdrawal of the catheter by 3 cm and a further 15 mL eventually produced a satisfactory block for surgery.

Epidurogram findings: midline septum with lateral extensions

Anteroposterior screening revealed the first 9 mL of contrast to be entirely on the right side from L2–S1 (Fig. 7.6a, p.92). The catheter tip appeared to be at L3 just to the right of the midline. The following 4 mL spread

to the left, to fill a dense restricted mass from L2 to L4. The AP radiograph (Fig. 7.6a) shows the predominantly right unilateral spread, with the suggestion of a straight midline border from L3 to S1, and mainly right-sided foraminal spill. In the lateral aspect (Fig. 7.6b) there were marked anterior and posterior columns of contrast, with a large central filling defect between. This middle zone was almost completely free of contrast above L5. The combined images are suggestive of a lumbar dorsal midline septum, with a broad lateral extension

89

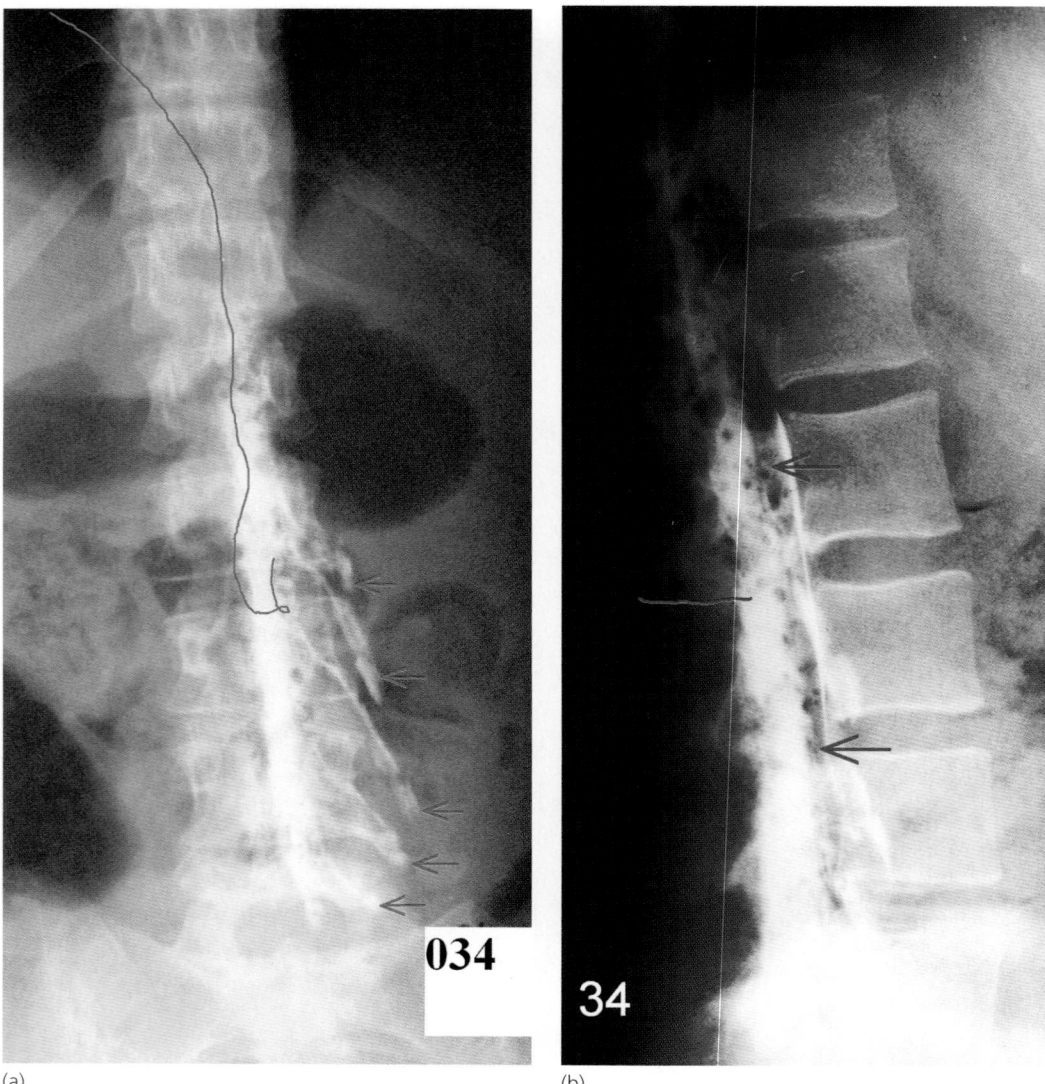

(a)   (b)

● **Fig. 7.5** (a) Anteroposterior (AP) epidurogram with catheter-tip at L2–3 and almost totally left-sided spread of contrast from L1 to L5 and profuse left foraminal spill (arrowed). Appearances suggestive of a midline septum. (b) Lateral epidurogram following unilateral block. There is a restricted spread of contrast from L1 to L5, with a pronounced posterior column of epidural contrast containing air bubbles. The attenuated anterior column of contrast is separated by a central filling defect (arrowed), suggesting the presence of a transverse septum in addition to the midline septum.

producing the central filling defect, and the catheter tip (O) positioned in the right posterior dorsolateral space (Fig. 7.6c).

The unusual features of this case were the recurring nature of the right unilateral block in successive pregnancies, and the late spread of contrast to the unblocked side. The value of screening is clearly demonstrated here, as the AP radiograph does not disclose the totally unilateral initial distribution of contrast.

7.5.3 The transverse septum

Three examples of an obstructive transverse septum are described in Case Histories 7.5–7.7. The clinical presentation

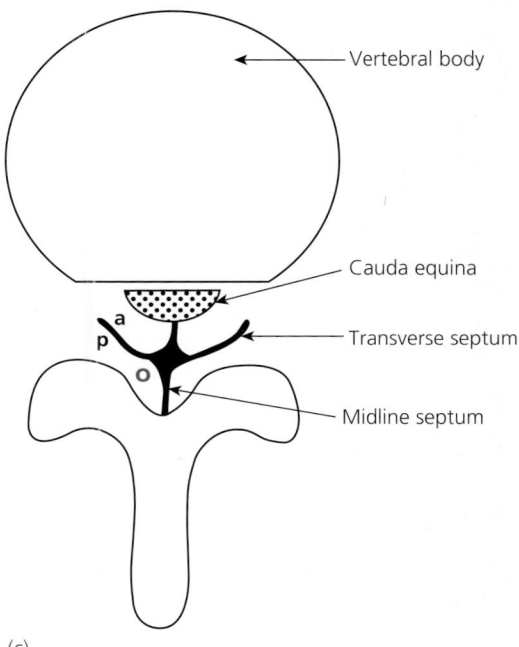

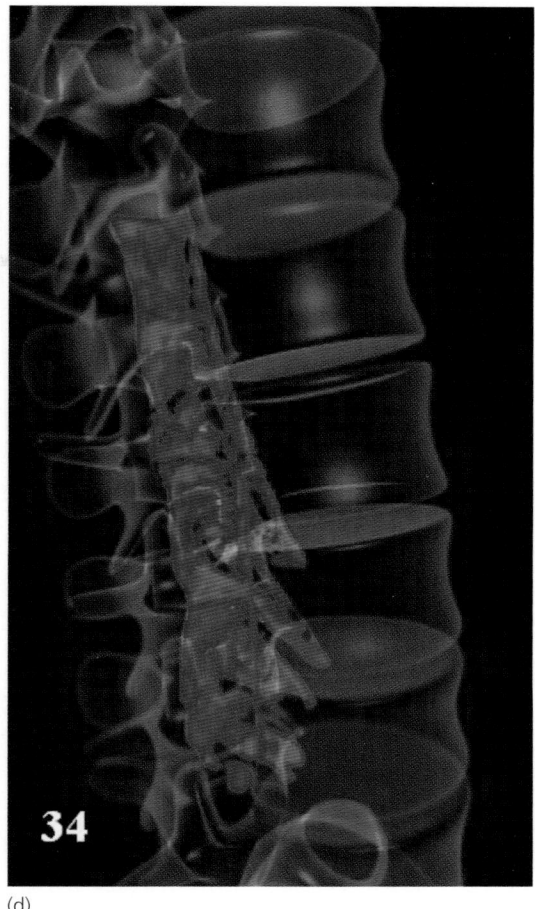

34

(c) (d)

● **Fig. 7.5** (Continued) (c) Diagram of septal anatomy and presumed position of catheter tip (O) in the left posterior dorsolateral space. (d) A three-dimensional model of the unilateral mass of contrast (oblique view) showing profuse left-sided foraminal spill.

was of an 'incomplete block', defined here as an epidural block with initial lack of vertical spread and exhibiting persistent failure to extend high enough or low enough, or occasionally both. The injected local anaesthetic appears to be predominantly confined behind the septum, at least initially, and has limited access to its sites of action.

CASE HISTORY 7.5:
INCOMPLETE BLOCK OF SACRAL ROOTS

In a labouring patient, initial epidural block at L3–4, using a 'closer-eye' catheter (Portex) inserted to 4 cm within the epidural space, produced bilateral block from T9 to L5 but no sacral analgesia, despite repeated doses of local anaesthetic over 2 h, totalling 40 mL lidocaine 2% with adrenaline. The catheter was removed and subsequent block at L2–3 with a further 15 mL dose raised the

sensory level to T4, but with only poor sacral block developing.

Epidurogram findings: transverse septum
Screening of the AP epidurogram showed that the catheter tip was at L2 in the midline and bilateral contrast was spread extensively from T5 to S1, with an unusual epidural appearance in that there was minimal foraminal spill and no lateral columns of contrast. The AP radiograph (Fig. 7.7a) shows a fairly dense central body of contrast from T10 to L2 (red arrows) that is fairly amorphous, but with scalloped edges. Above and below the main body, from T5 to T10 and L2 to S1, the contrast becomes patchy and attenuated, with multiple filling defects and air bubbles. The overall appearance suggests that the contrast is predominantly at the back of the epidural space.

91

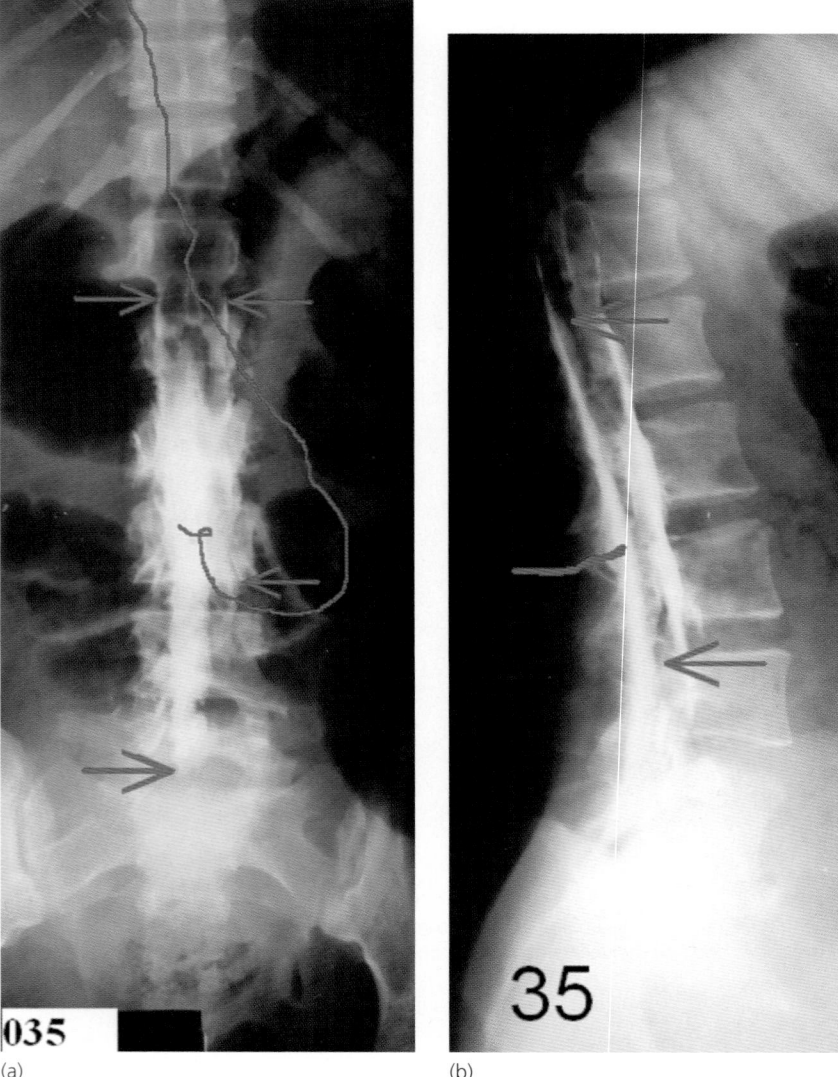

(a)   (b)

● **Fig. 7.6** (a) Anteroposterior (AP) epidurogram with predominantly right-sided contrast spread from L1 to S1 (arrowed), with prominent right foraminal spill and a straight medial border between L3 and S1. Appearances suggest a midline septum. (b) Lateral epidurogram in the same patient, with marked anterior and posterior columns of contrast from L5 to S1, enclosing a large filling defect (arrowed), suggesting a transverse septum, in addition to a midline septum.

The lateral view (Fig. 7.7b) confirms that most of the contrast had indeed flowed posteriorly, with a dense posterior column (blue arrows). There was minimal contrast anteriorly where the anterior column usually appears, just a number of filling defects (red arrows), interspersed with numerous air bubbles. The presence of a fairly broad transverse septum is presumed. The bilateral filling of the posterior epidural space suggests that any midline structure attached to the transverse

septum is probably rudimentary and non-obstructive, suggesting that there is no effective midline septum in this case (Fig. 7.7c).

While it is thought that the presence of excessive volumes of air bubbles in the epidural space can possibly impede the action of local anaesthetic agents,[10,11] it does seem to be an unlikely explanation in this case (and the next two) even though the sacral roots can be notoriously difficult to block and the loss of resistance

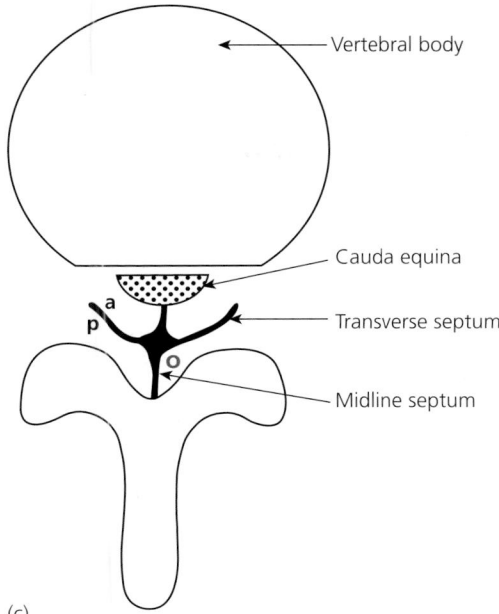

(c)

● **Fig. 7.6** (Continued) (c) Diagram of septal anatomy and presumed position of catheter tip (O) in the right posterior dorsolateral space.

to air test was used twice (two catheter insertions). It is more likely that the posterior distribution of the contrast was the significant factor, for if this represented spread of the local anaesthetic then little would have reached far enough anteriorly to reach the nerve roots at the intervertebral foramina, especially in the lower lumbar and sacral areas.

CASE HISTORY 7.6:
INCOMPLETE BLOCK, LIMITED SPREAD

A labouring patient received an epidural puncture at L3–4, using a three lateral eye catheter (Portex) inserted to 4 cm, and developed a very limited bilateral block between T11 and L4. Upper abdominal pain persisted throughout early labour and no sacral block developed, despite five top-up doses of lidocaine 2% with adrenaline, total 60 mL, being given over 6 h.

Epidurogram findings: **transverse septum**
The AP epidurogram (Fig. 7.8a) shows the catheter tip in the midline at L3. The contrast appearance is very similar to the previous case, showing contrast from T10 to L5. Again, there is a dense amorphous central body of contrast with scalloped edges containing numerous air

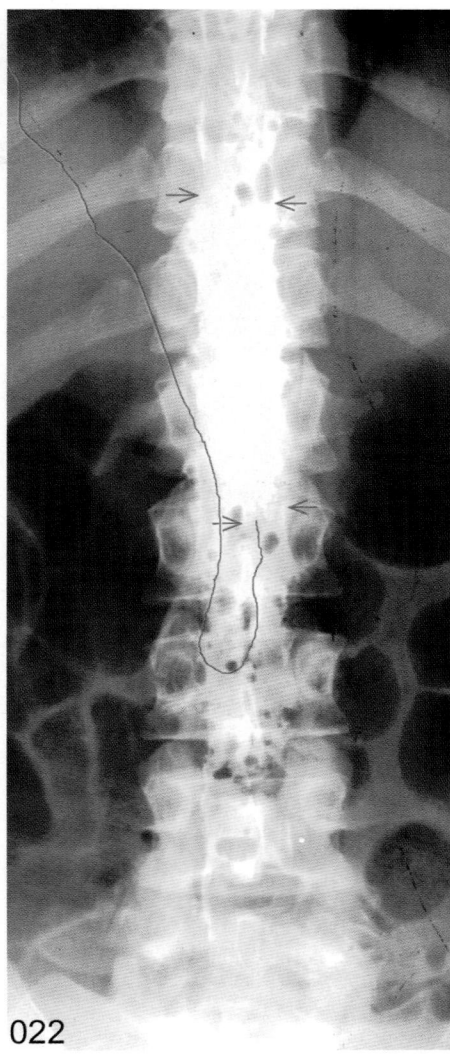

022

(a)

● **Fig. 7.7** (a) Anteroposterior (AP) epidurogram showing fairly extensive contrast spread from T5 to S1, with a dense collection from T11 to L2 (arrowed), which has characteristic scalloped edges and suggests a posterior distribution of contrast. There is minimal foraminal spill.

bubbles and extending from L1 to L4 (red arrows). Above and below the main body, between T10 and L1 and L4 and L5, the contrast becomes patchy and attenuated, with multiple filling defects and air bubbles. There is minimal foraminal spill and no lateral columns.

The lateral view (Fig. 7.8b) displays the marked posterior distribution of the contrast (blue arrows), with a

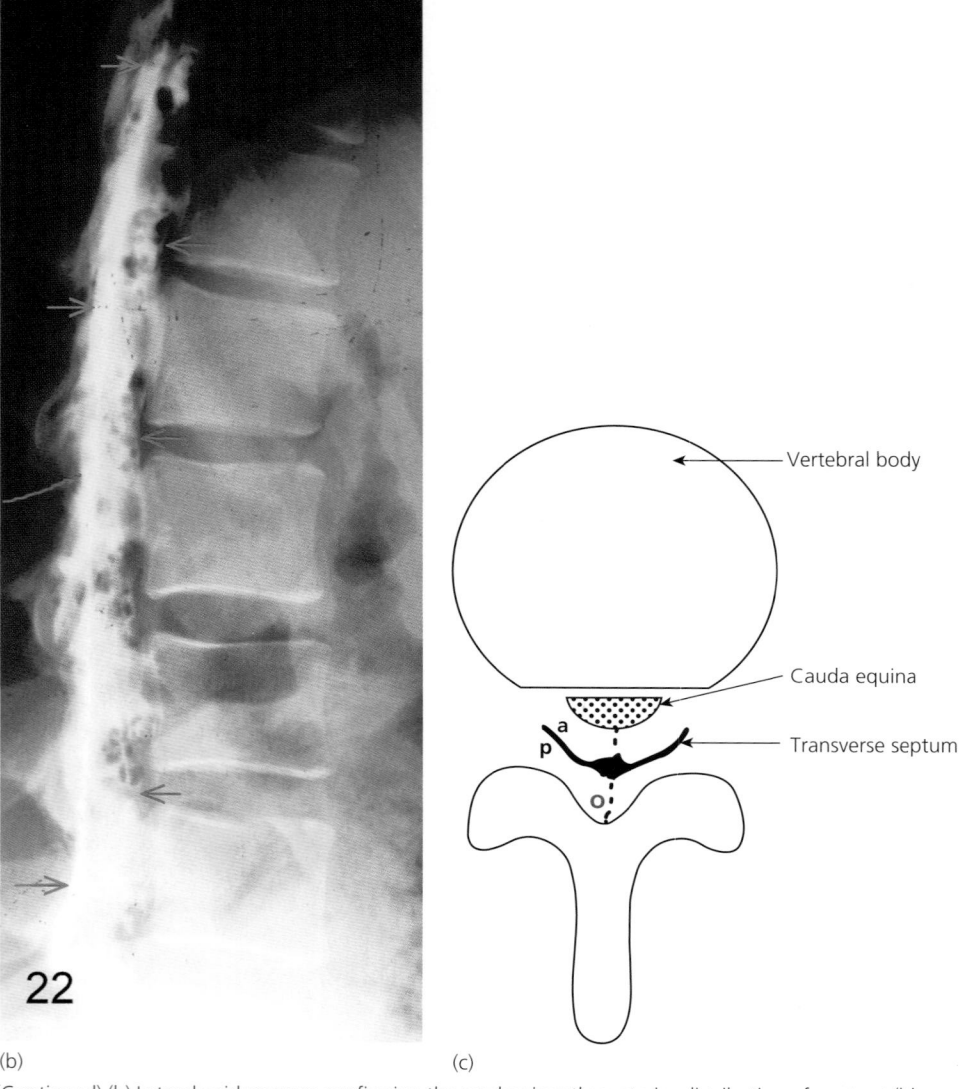

(b)   (c)

● **Fig. 7.7** (Continued) (b) Lateral epidurogram confirming the predominantly posterior distribution of contrast (blue arrows), with absent anterior column and multiple filling defects (red arrows) containing air bubbles and only sparse contrast. Combined images suggest the presence of a transverse septum. (c) Diagram of septal anatomy and presumed position of the catheter tip (O) in the posterior dorsolateral space.

very attenuated and fragmented anterior column present. The large central filling defect (red arrows) contains only small patches of contrast and numerous air bubbles. The combined images suggest the presence of a transverse septum, with no significant midline component, as shown in Fig. 7.7c.

CASE HISTORY 7.7:

LOW ASYMMETRIC BLOCK, FAILED POSTOPERATIVE ANALGESIA

A 47-year-old patient received an L2–3 epidural block, with 4 cm of catheter being left in the epidural space, prior

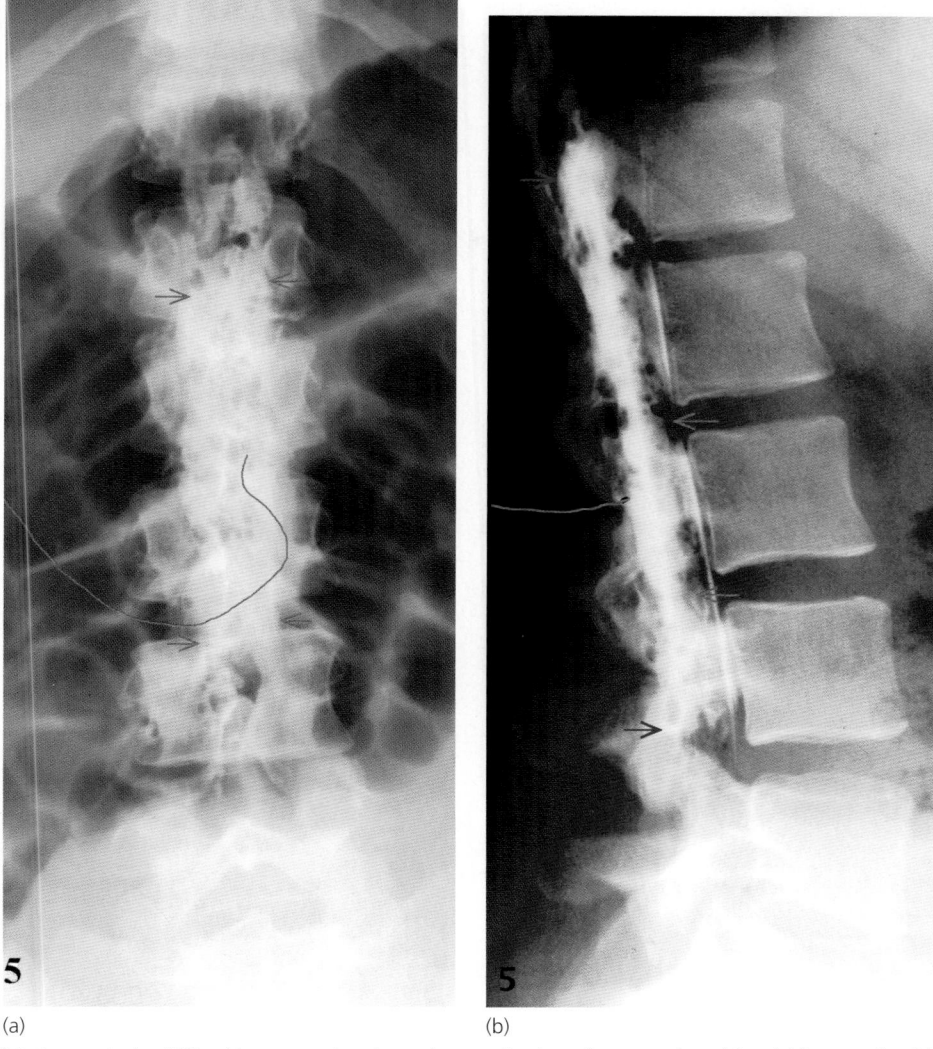

(a)   (b)

● **Fig. 7.8** (a) Anteroposterior (AP) epidurogram showing a dense collection of contrast from L1 to L4 (arrowed), with characteristic scalloped edges and minimal foraminal spill, predominantly at the back of the epidural space. (b) Lateral epidurogram confirming the predominantly posterior distribution of contrast (blue arrows), with very attenuated anterior column and large filling defect (red arrows) containing air bubbles in a sparse mass of contrast. The combined images suggest the presence of a transverse septum.

to general anaesthesia for abdominal hysterectomy. The catheter was a 19 gauge, wire-reinforced type (Arrow) with a terminal hole, and directed cephalad. The block level prior to surgery was only at T10, following 20 mL lidocaine 2%, and the left foot remained cold throughout, suggesting poor left lumbar sympathetic block. A postoperative epidural infusion of bupivacaine/fentanyl produced inadequate analgesia, and an epidurogram was undertaken the following day.

Epidurogram findings: transverse septum

Screening revealed the catheter tip to be at L3 in the midline, and directed caudally. On injection, contrast was seen to collect centrally at L2–3, then spread caudally to L5 and finally cephalad to T4. The AP epidurogram (Fig. 7.9a) confirms the extensive spread of contrast from T4 to L5, with a 'fusiform' appearance that starts to taper off at T11 above and L4 below. As in the two previous cases, there are many small filling defects in the

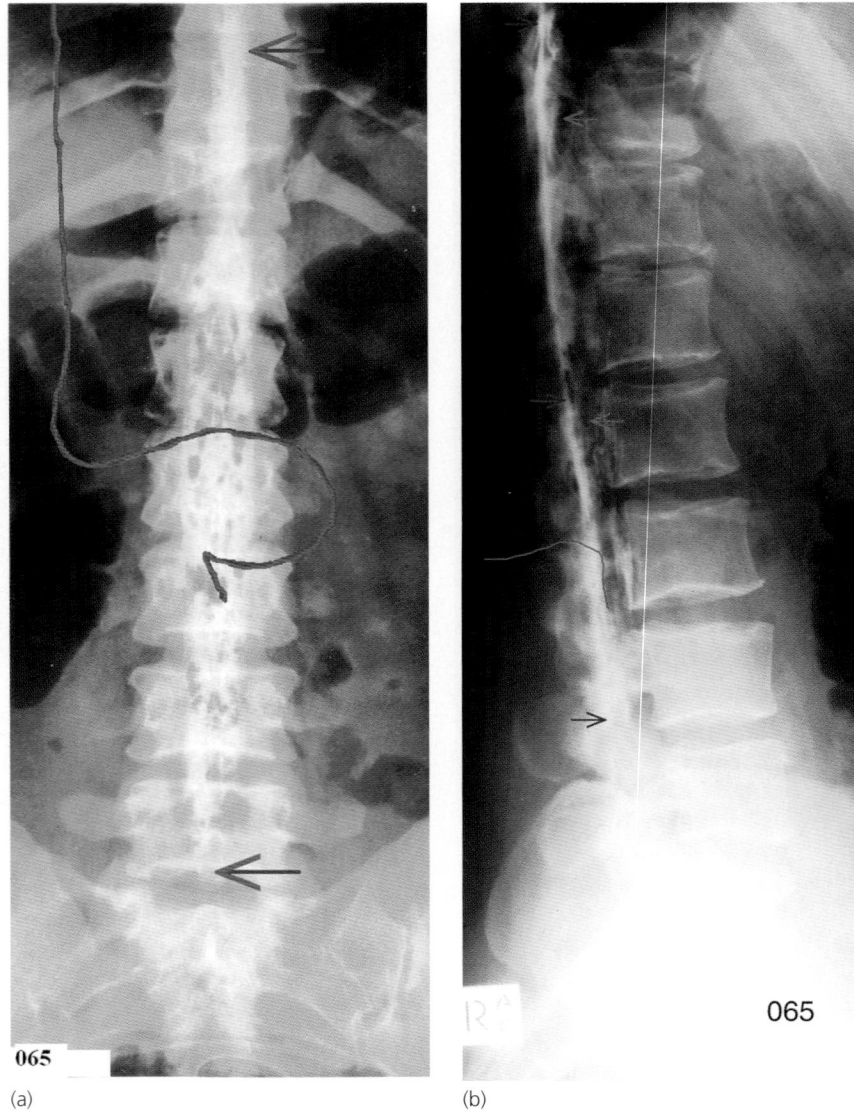

(a)   (b)

● **Fig. 7.9** (a) Anteroposterior (AP) epidurogram revealing catheter tip pointing caudally, with extensive but narrow spread of contrast in a characteristic 'fusiform' shape suggestive of posterior distribution, from T5 to L5 (arrows), with a smooth outline and containing air bubbles. (b) Lateral epidurogram confirming the predominantly posterior distribution of contrast (blue arrows), with only a very attenuated anterior column, at L2, and a large filling defect (red arrows) containing air bubbles and sparse contrast. Combined images suggest the presence of a transverse septum, at the very back of the epidural space.

main body of contrast, with no lateral columns and no foraminal spill, but the contrast outline is smooth, rather than scalloped. The lateral view (Fig. 7.9b) displays the marked posterior distribution of the contrast (blue arrows), with a very short attenuated anterior column present at L3. The large anterior filling defect (red arrows) contains only small patches of contrast and a few air bubbles. A transverse septum appears to be the most likely diagnosis.

The fusiform appearance of the contrast, with its smooth outline, has been noted on two other occasions, and it appears to result from the transverse septum being located towards the back of the epidural space – further back than was evident in the previous two cases.

With these three cases involving a transverse septum, it seems reasonable to surmise that the tips of the epidural

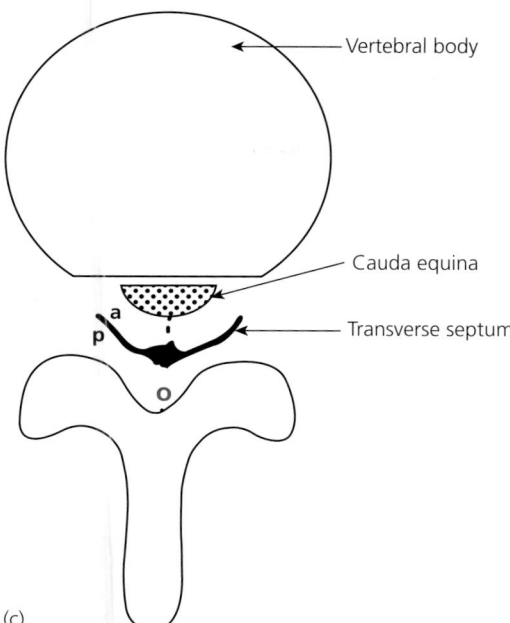

Vertebral body

Cauda equina

Transverse septum

(c)

● **Fig. 7.9** (Continued) (c) Diagram of septal anatomy and presumed position of catheter tip (O) in the posterior dorsolateral space, with no midline septum.

catheters were positioned in the posterior compartment of the dorsolateral epidural space, but in the absence of a significant midline septum, as flow across the midline was seen to be unrestricted. The midline septum may be rudimentary as shown in Fig. 7.7c or absent as in Fig. 7.9c. It appears that the restricted epidural spread of local anaesthetic caused by a transverse septum may usually be overcome, at least partly, by increasing the volume injected, when leakage out of the posterior 'compartment' will probably occur.

7.6 Conclusions

This chapter has included a description of three different types of septal barrier which may impede the free flow of solutions in the epidural space, and which account for just over half of our cases of failed blocks. Whether obstruction results from a true midline septum, a true transverse septum or a hybrid structure, a failed or inadequate block may result. We estimate that the incidence of a significant septum in our parturients is approximately 3%, and some of these patients will require a second epidural catheter, at a different interspace, for a successful result. There appears to be a clear role for epidurography in the elucidation of unilateral

and other inadequate blocks, as they may recur on future occasions.

REFERENCES

1 Blomberg RG (1986) The dorsomedian connective tissue band in the lumbar epidural space of humans. An anatomical study using epiduroscopy in autopsy cases. *Anesthesia and Analgesia*; 65:747–752.
2 Savolaine ER, Pandya JB, Greenblatt SH, Conover SR (1988) Anatomy of the lumbar epidural space: New insights using CT-epidurography. *Anesthesiology*; 68:217–220.
3 Hogan QH, Lynch K, Lacitis I (1993) Histologic features of epidural soft tissue and its relation to the dura and canal wall. *Regional Anesthesia*; 18(2S):54.
4 Hogan QH (1999) Epidural catheter tip position and distribution of injectate evaluated by computed tomography. *Anesthesiology*; 90:964–970.
5 Hatten HP (1980) Lumbar epidurography with metrizamide. *Radiology*; 137:129–136.
6 Seeling W, Tomczak R, Merk J, Mrakovcić N (1995) Comparison of conventional and computed tomographic epidurography with contrast medium using thoracic epidural catheters. *Anaesthetist*; 44:24–36.
7 Hogan QH (1991) Lumbar epidural anatomy. A new look by cryomicrotome section. *Anesthesiology*; 75:767–775.
8 Gaynor A (1990) The lumbar epidural region: Anatomy and approach. In *Epidural and Spinal Blockade in Obstetrics*, editor Reynolds F. Balliere Tindall, London, pp. 1–18.
9 Capogna G, Celleno D, Simonetti C, Lupoi D (1997) Anatomy of the lumbar epidural region using magnetic resonance imaging: a study of dimensions and a comparison of two postures. *International Journal of Obstetric Anesthesia*; 6:97–100.
10 Boezaart AP, Levendig BJ (1989) Epidural air-filled bubbles and unblocked segments. *Canadian Journal of Anaesthesia*; 36:603–604.
11 Dalens B, Bazin J, Haberer J (1987) Epidural bubbles as a cause of incomplete analgesia during epidural anesthesia. *Anesthesia and Analgesia*; 66:679–683.

CHAPTER 8
SPINAL DEFORMITY AND EPIDURAL BLOCK

Patients with marked spinal deformity, whether congenital or acquired, may be expected to present with technically difficult or impossible epidural needle or catheter insertion. The resulting blocks, if attained, are often patchy and inadequate. Lesser degrees of deformity may also be associated with unsatisfactory or unusually extensive blocks. The deformities described in regard to epidural block in this chapter are:

1 Scoliosis
2 Kyphosis and lordosis
3 Spinal pathology/spinal surgery
4 Congenital block vertebrae
5 Spina bifida occulta

One notable failed epidural block from many years ago, involved a patient with an extreme degree of congenital kyphoscoliosis as shown in Fig. 8.1. Neither the epidural, caudal nor the subarachnoid spaces could be located in this pregnant patient, despite the efforts of several 'experts'. As she also had very limited mouth-opening, and could not be intubated, her elective caesarean section was performed under infiltration local anaesthesia, with only minor discomfort.

8.1 Scoliosis

For many years, significant cases of scoliosis have been treated with corrective surgery in adolescence. Harrington rod instrumentation was the usual management in our scoliosis patients (Fig. 8.2) but this operation has been superseded, and we are now seeing the last of these patients as they reach their child-bearing days. Current surgical techniques are less invasive and may involve an anterior release with posterior segmental instrumentation and spinal fusion.[1]

We anticipated unsatisfactory epidural blocks in patients with marked scoliosis,[1] particularly in those who had undergone spinal surgery.[2] However, we were surprised to find that even minor degrees of scoliosis, of which the patient was often unaware, were associated with blocks that were 'patchy' and frequently unilateral, at least initially,

especially when low concentrations of local anaesthetic were being used in labour. On several occasions a second epidural catheter in an adjacent interspace was required for satisfactory block,[3] or a subarachnoid block introduced.[4]

Once the scoliosis was detected during a post-partum radiograph, the patient would often recall scoliosis being

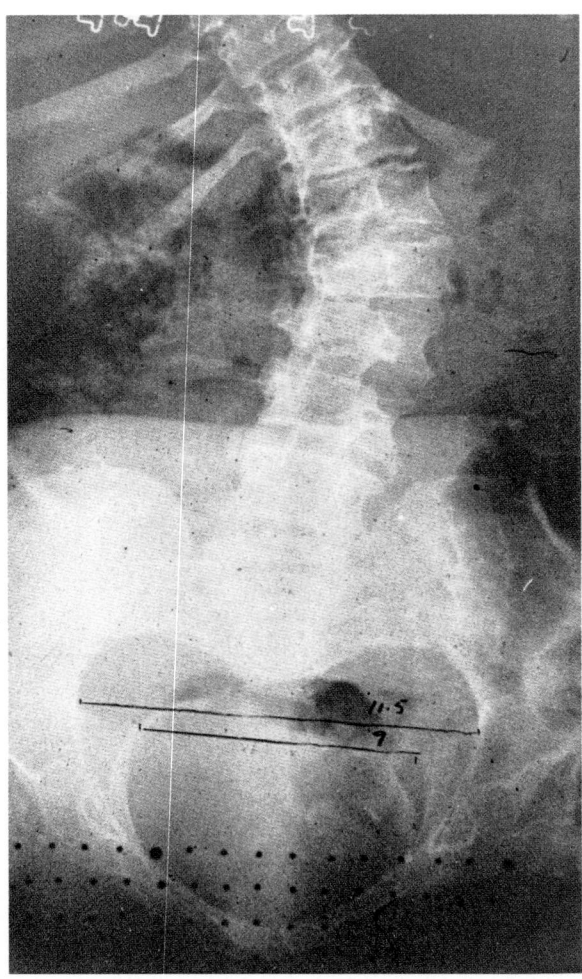

● **Fig. 8.1** Anteroposterior (AP) radiograph (from 1974) used for pelvimetry. Severe kyphoscoliosis is noted, and the presence of a term foetal head *in utero*.

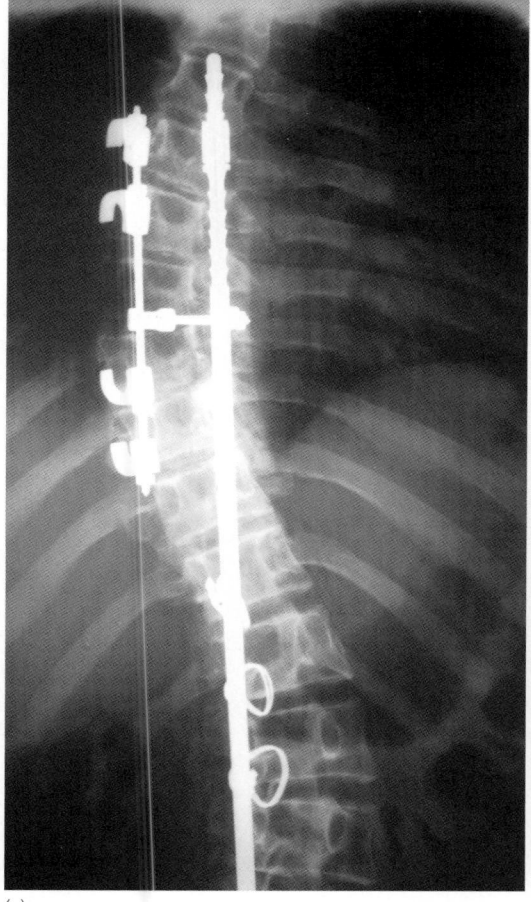

(a)

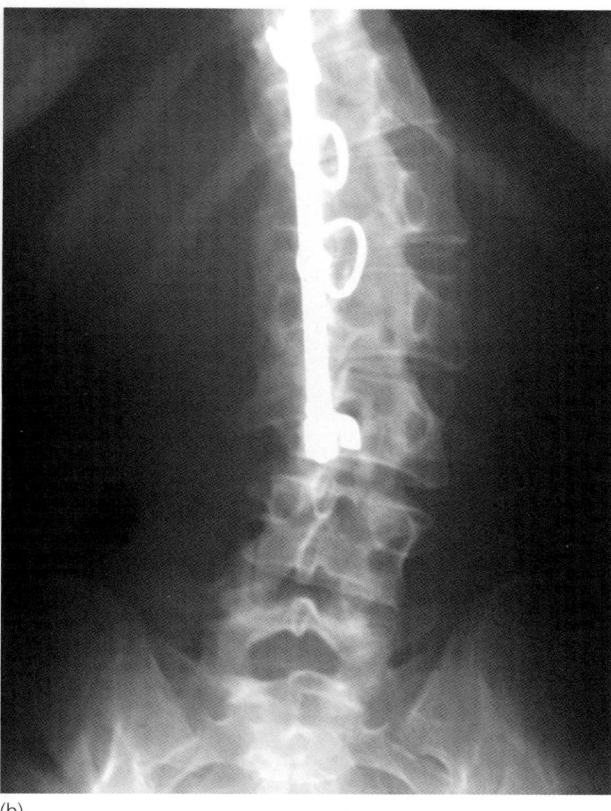

(b)

● **Fig. 8.2** (a) Anteroposterior (AP) radiograph of familial scoliosis with Harrington rod instrumentation, upper view. (b) An AP radiograph of familial scoliosis with Harrington rod instrumentation, lower view, with presence of spina bifida occulta (SBO) at S1.

diagnosed at a school doctor's examination many years before. Scoliosis did appear to a major factor in disrupting satisfactory epidural blocks, as it occurred in 23% of our study group of 100 pregnant patients with failed or inadequate blocks, representing the second most common cause of failure in this series, after obstruction by a septum.

CASE HISTORY 8.1:
PERSISTENT UNILATERAL BLOCK

A 29-year-old patient was unaware of any spinal deformity prior to her epidural block in labour, and had never suffered any back problems. The anaesthetist did not detect any deformity when performing the epidural. A persistent right-sided block developed, following a straightforward epidural puncture at L2–3 and an injection of 5 mL bupivacaine 0.375% through a Tuohy needle, followed by another 15 mL through a closer-eye

catheter (Portex), which was inserted to a depth of 3 cm in the epidural space. Good analgesia up to T9 developed on the right after 10 min without motor block, but the left side was totally unblocked, even after a further bolus of 6 mL was injected in the lateral position. Repeat puncture at L3–4, with the addition of 16 mL lidocaine 2%, produced no improvement and intramuscular analgesia was required. This was one of the few cases studied where neither repeated volumes of local anaesthetic nor contrast appeared to cross the midline to the unaffected side in a significant volume.

Epidurogram findings: scoliosis, predominantly unilateral contrast

The anteroposterior (AP) epidurogram (Fig. 8.3a) following delivery shows a fairly minor degree of thoracolumbar scoliosis with a primary curve convex to the left. Rotation of the lower thoracic spinous processes

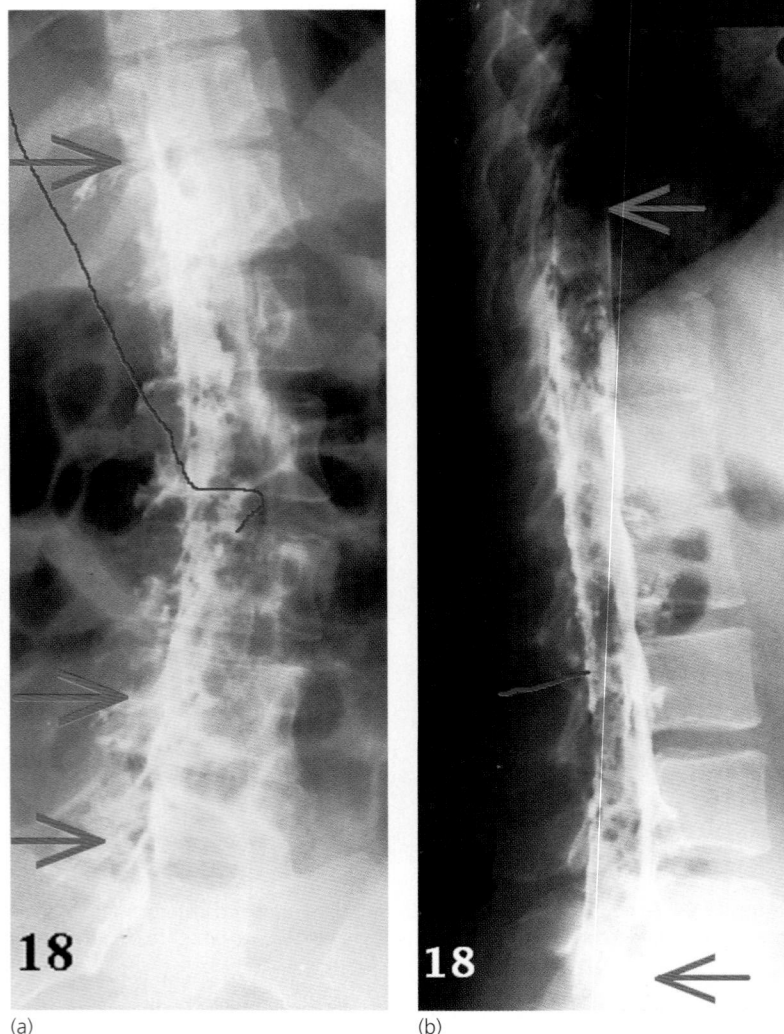

(a) (b)

● **Fig. 8.3** (a) Anteroposterior (AP) epidurogram with mild scoliosis. The contrast is predominantly right-sided from T10 to S1 with profuse right-sided transforaminal spill (arrowed) and only patchy left-sided contrast from T10 to L2. (b) Lateral epidurogram showing a loss of lumbar lordosis, with patchy spread of contrast across the lower thoracolumbar epidural space (arrowed).

is clearly visible. The tip of the epidural catheter can be seen at L4, just to the right of midline, pointing caudally, although it had been directed rostrally. The contrast is mostly confined to the right side of the vertebral canal, with good foraminal spill between T10 and the sacrum (arrowed). On the left side, there is a small volume of patchy contrast between T10 and L2, but no foraminal spill.

The lateral view (Fig. 8.3b) shows a very straight lumbar spine, with loss of the usual lordosis, and fairly uniform contrast filling across the right side of the epidural space (arrowed), although the posterior column of contrast is a little patchy in places. It seems likely that the spinal curvature of scoliosis is mainly responsible for the maldistribution of epidural solutions in this patient, favouring the inside of the scoliotic curve. However, the scoliosis may also have contributed to the caudal displacement of the catheter tip, as well as its displacement to the inside of the curve (in this case, the right), which is a relatively common finding.

CASE HISTORY 8.2:
RECURRING UNILATERAL BLOCK

A 36-year-old patient in her first labour received an epidural block at L2–3, using a three lateral eye catheter (Portex), inserted uneventfully to a depth of 4 cm within the epidural space. There was no history of scoliosis or back problems. The block remained totally right-sided, despite the administration of 40 mL of bupivacaine 0.125% over 2 h. On inspection, the skin dressing over the epidural site was noted to be saturated with fluid. The epidural catheter was removed and reinserted in the same space. A further dose of 15 mL, given through the Tuohy needle, produced satisfactory bilateral block for 90 min. After that time, an infusion provided only right-sided block. An epidurogram was undertaken on the following day.

Epidurogram findings; scoliosis, unilateral contrast

On AP fluoroscopic screening, the catheter tip was seen to be in the midline at L3. A mild degree of scoliosis was noted, with the lumbar curve to the left and rotation of several lower thoracic vertebral bodies (Fig. 8.4a). The AP epidurogram reveals totally right-sided contrast from T10 to L5 (arrowed). The lateral view (Fig. 8.4b) shows an increased lumbar lordosis, with uniform spread of contrast across (the right side of) the lumbar epidural space (arrowed), with clearly defined anterior and posterior columns. Above L2, there is no anterior column.

These first two cases represent almost totally unilateral blocks, probably directly attributable to the presence of scoliosis. Retrograde flow of contrast around the outside of the catheter, to either the erector spinae muscles or skin, was commonly seen in cases of unilateral block, whenever there was obstruction to inward flow of contrast (see Fig. 6.8c, p.81). Case History 8.3 appears to have the combined problems of scoliosis and a coexisting midline septum.

CASE HISTORY 8.3:
PERSISTENT UNILATERAL BLOCK

A 36-year-old patient in her first labour underwent epidural block at L3–4, with uneventful insertion of 4 cm of a closer-eye catheter (Portex) into the epidural space. She gave no history of back problems or scoliosis. She did not develop satisfactory analgesia on her left side, throughout a 10-h labour, despite repeated doses of bupivacaine 0.375%, to a total of 60 mL. When an urgent caesarean section was scheduled, general anaesthesia was induced.

Epidurogram findings: spinal deformity, scoliosis, with probable septum

On AP fluoroscopic screening the following day, a mild degree of scoliosis was noted, with the catheter tip at L3–4 just to the right of the midline (Fig. 8.5a). Administration of contrast was difficult as there was considerable resistance to injection and it took over 90 s to insert a 10 mL volume. Contrast appeared initially only on the right side, with a straight midline border and foraminal spill after 45 s. By 90 s, a small volume of contrast had flowed to the left, from T10 downwards. The AP epidurogram (Fig. 8.5a) shows the mild scoliosis with a primary thoracolumbar curve to the left. Rotation of the lower thoracic spinous processes is clearly visible. Right-sided contrast is seen from T8 to L5, with abundant foraminal spill (red arrows). On the left side there is a small body of contrast at T10–T11, which spreads to a very narrow lateral column down to L3 (blue arrows). The lateral view (Fig. 8.5b) was of poor quality, but there was seen to be fairly uniform spread of contrast across the lumbar epidural space (arrowed), or at least the right side of the space, with a high posterior column. It seems likely that the scoliosis contributed to the maldistribution of the contrast, but the possible role of a coexisting midline septum must be considered, in view of the straight midline border seen on screening.

On reviewing the epidurograms of six other patients with similar scoliotic deformity, the most distinctive feature was the predominantly unilateral spread of contrast away from the primary convex spinal curve, (contrast tends to flow towards the inside of the curve), mirroring the spread of the preceding nerve-block, although this was not invariable. Additional doses of local anaesthetic will sometimes correct a failed block caused by scoliosis, otherwise the addition of a second epidural catheter may be necessary. We have found it to be advantageous to insert the second catheter, in an adjacent interspace, using a paramedian approach to the epidural space, from the unblocked side.

8.2 Kyphosis and lordosis

Although kyphosis, lordosis and scoliosis frequently coexist, particularly in the elderly, they may also be found in isolation. Kyphotic or lordotic deformities alone have not specifically been associated with any failed or inadequate blocks in this work, but extensive cephalad spread of epidural solutions did occur with both deformities. In addition, marked degrees of lumbar lordosis did make epidural insertion more difficult,

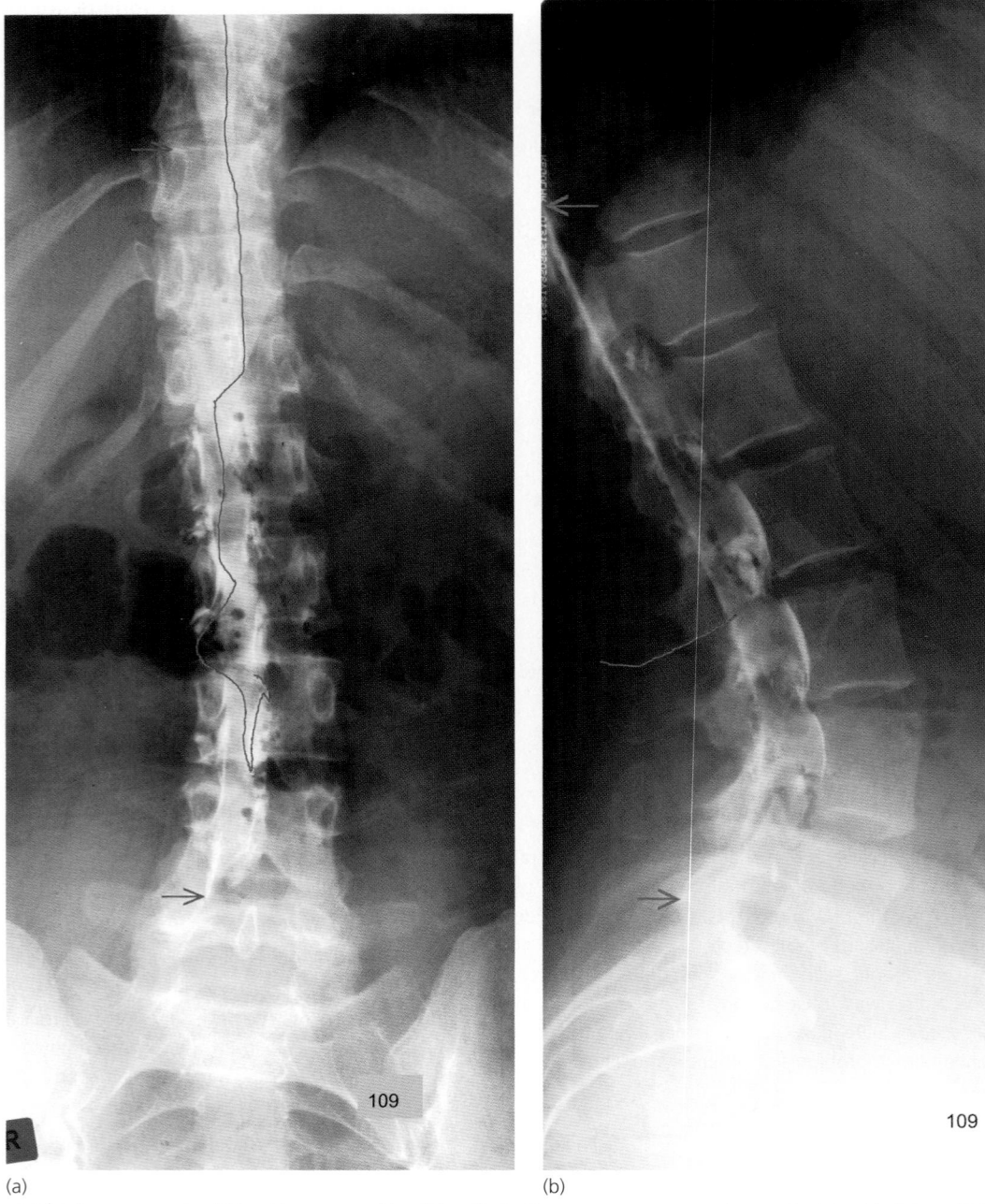

(a)   (b)

● **Fig. 8.4** (a) Anteroposterior (AP) epidurogram with mild scoliosis. The contrast appears to be totally right-sided, from T10 to L5, (arrowed) with right-sided transforaminal spill. (b) Lateral epidurogram showing an increased lumbar lordosis. There is faint, but fairly uniform spread of contrast across the lumbar epidural space (arrowed), but the anterior column of contrast does not extend above L2.

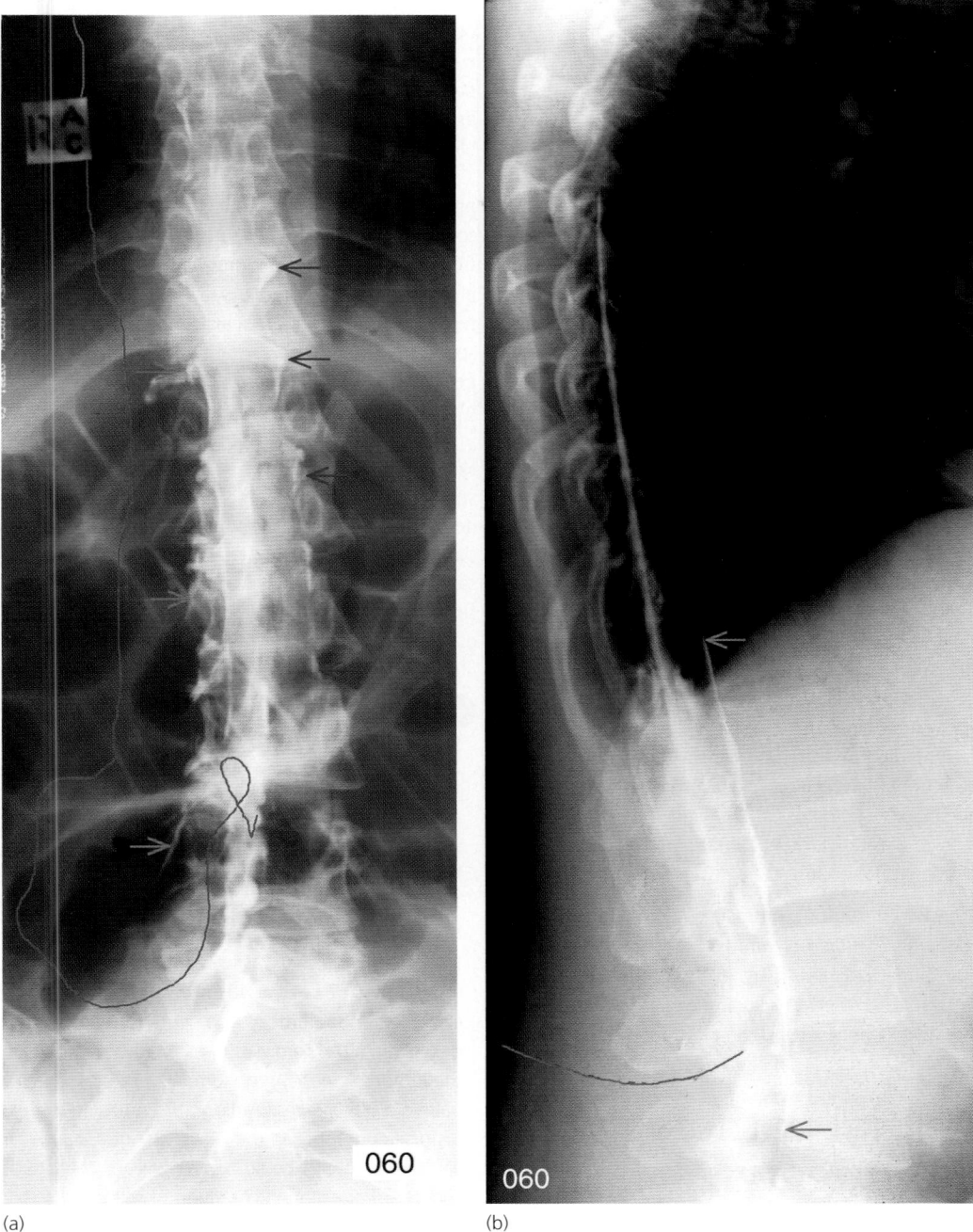

(a)   (b)

● **Fig. 8.5** (a) Anteroposterior (AP) epidurogram with mild scoliosis. The contrast is mostly right-sided from T8 to L5 with a fairly straight midline border. There is profuse right-sided transforaminal spill (red arrows). Sparse left-sided contrast spread from T10 to L3 is present, with a narrow lateral column (blue arrows). (b) Lateral epidurogram in the presence of scoliosis. There is a uniform spread of contrast across the lumbar epidural space (arrowed), with an extensive posterior column above.

SPINAL DEFORMITY AND EPIDURAL BLOCK

with a higher failure rate in the hands of inexperienced personnel.

CASE HISTORY 8.4:
HIGH SENSORY BLOCK

A 66-year-old patient with a marked kyphosis presented for epidural block prior to gynaecological surgery in the lithotomy position. Her degree of spinal curvature was so great that three pillows were required to support her head and neck in a comfortable position. Following straightforward epidural puncture at L2–3, a lateral eye catheter (Portex) was inserted to a depth of 3 cm and 16 mL lidocaine 1.5% injected. The block was adequate for surgery after 20 min, but the sensory level continued to rise, reaching T2 after 40 min, with only a minimal fall in blood pressure and no respiratory difficulty.

Epidurogram findings: **kyphosis with high posterior contrast column**

The AP epidurogram (Fig. 8.6a) reveals marked degenerative change in the vertebral bodies and the extensive but patchy spread of epidural contrast from T2 to L5, with an irregular, scalloped outline. There is extensive foraminal spill, producing an unusual 'cauliflower' appearance at several levels (arrowed). The lower part of the lateral view displays a typical pattern of contrast spreading uniformly across the lumbar epidural space. The upper lateral view (Fig. 8.6b) reveals the anterior column terminating at L1, while the posterior column continues upwards to T2 (arrowed) following the curve of the kyphotic spine.

An extensive posterior contrast column, following a high sensory block, was a common finding in our older gynaecological patients. It is difficult to determine whether this was attributable solely to a kyphotic curve, or partly due to degenerative changes restricting outflow through the intervertebral foramina.

8.3 Spinal pathology/ spinal surgery

Fortunately, times have changed since many neurosurgeons and orthopaedic surgeons actively discouraged their patients with major back problems from receiving epidural or spinal blocks for labour, caesarean section or other abdominal operations, even many years after spinal surgery, for fear of damaging their handiwork, injuring the spinal cord or nerve roots and exacerbating previous back symptoms. However, a similar situation appears to still exist in some cases of acute disc prolapse where many clinicians successfully employ

epidural block for pain relief, while others are vehemently opposed to such practice, without any firm supporting evidence. It also seems fairly illogical to deny a labouring patient with acute disc prolapse the benefits of epidural analgesia, as sometimes transpires, although satisfactory blocks may occasionally prove a challenge.[3]

Postsurgical blocks may be difficult or impossible in the presence of rods, bars and bone grafts, and the epidural space may be partly, or rarely completely, obliterated by fibrous adhesions.[1] Epidural adhesions may result from bleeding into the epidural space during surgery and in the recovery period, or from leakage of disc substance into the space following an annular tear. However, with care and persistence, satisfactory results may occur, although patchy blocks are not uncommon.[5-7]

Three postsurgical examples are described in Case Histories 8.5–8.7, the first involving the condition of spondylolisthesis.[8] For comparison, a scan of the uncorrected deformity in another patient is included (Fig. 8.7). This particular patient underwent a caesarean section under satisfactory epidural block at L2–3, while awaiting her spinal surgery, and her imaging showed marked anterior slippage of L5 on S1.

CASE HISTORY 8.5:
SATISFACTORY BLOCK AFTER SPINAL FUSION

A 42-year-old patient presented for elective caesarean section in her first pregnancy, with a history of spinal fusion for severe L5–S1 spondylolisthesis at the age of 16 years (in Europe). She suffered only mild backaches during her pregnancy. She was reviewed in the third trimester, when she was noted to be of slight stature (height 1.50 m, weight 48 kg) with a marked kyphosis, extreme lumbar lordosis and acute forward angulation of the sacrum. There was dense midline scarring over the lumbar spine, and no lumbar vertebral spines were palpable. Fairly recent radiographs revealed the highly distorted anatomy. In the AP view (Fig. 8.8a) no lumbar vertebra below L1 could be recognized. The lateral image (Fig. 8.8b) did allow recognition of some lumbosacral anatomy, but there appeared to be extensive bone grafts or new bone formation behind L3–5 (arrowed). Ultrasound scanning of the back was difficult because of the extreme angulation of the lumbosacral spine and proved unhelpful.

Prior to surgery, a Tuohy needle was inserted in the midline at the lowest palpable intervertebral space and 5 cm of a terminal eye catheter (Arrow) inserted into the epidural space, with remarkable ease. The precise

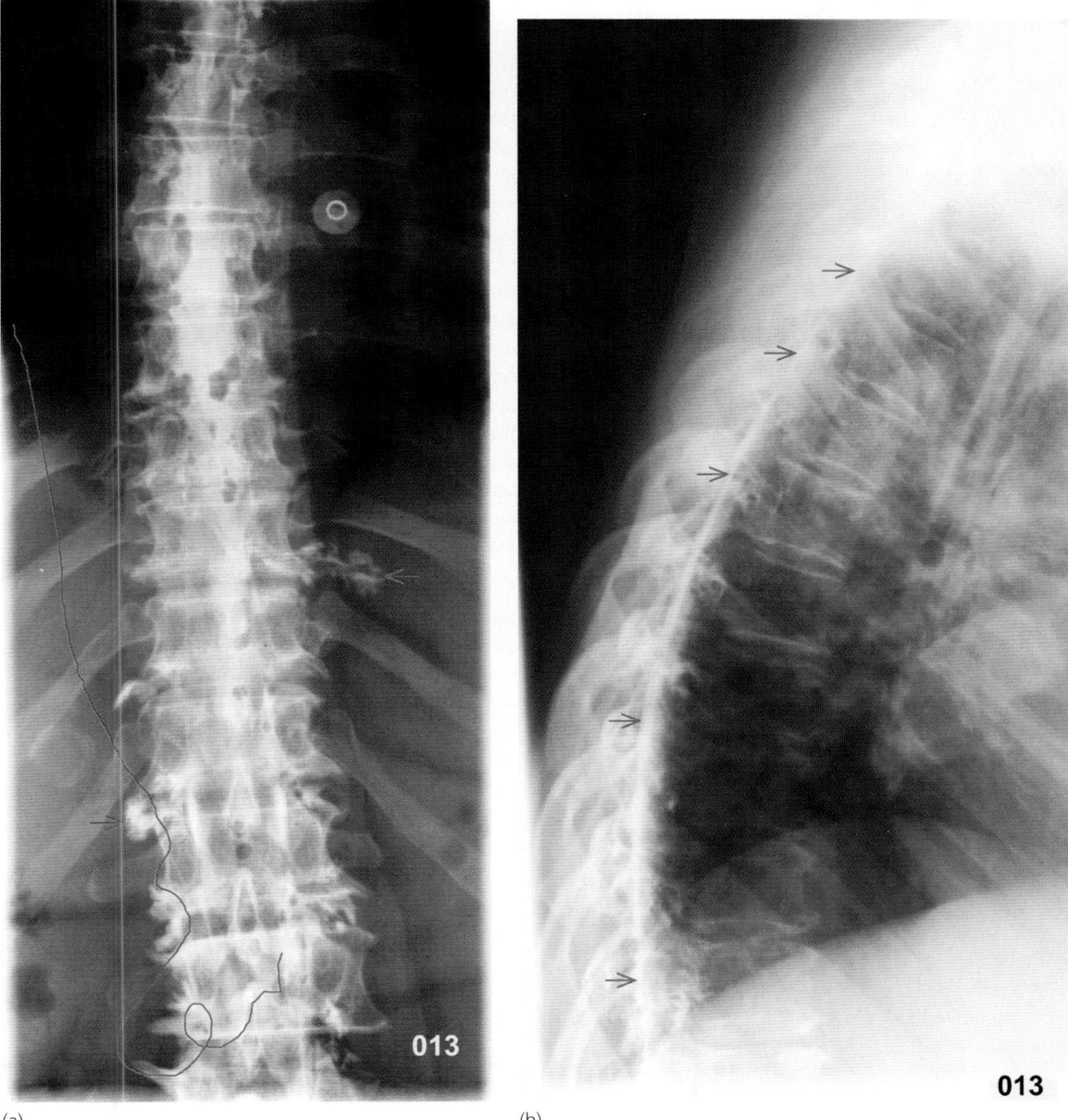

(a)   (b)

● **Fig. 8.6** (a) Anteroposterior (AP) epidurogram in an elderly patient with severe kyphosis. There is extensive but patchy spread of contrast from T2 to L5, with extensive transforaminal spill, which has an unusual 'cauliflower' appearance at several levels (arrowed). (b) Upper lateral epidurogram showing the severe kyphotic curve, with a very high posterior column of contrast (arrowed), extending to T2.

level of insertion could not be assessed, because of the distorted landmarks. The block from T3 to S2 was entirely satisfactory. An epidurogram was performed the following day, but contrast injection produced discomfort in the lower back, and was discontinued after 6 mL.

Epidurogram findings: thoracic contrast in typical distribution

On fluoroscopic screening, the epidural catheter was observed to have been inserted at T9–10, with the catheter tip in the midline and contrast flowing in a typical lateral column distribution from T5 to T11. The

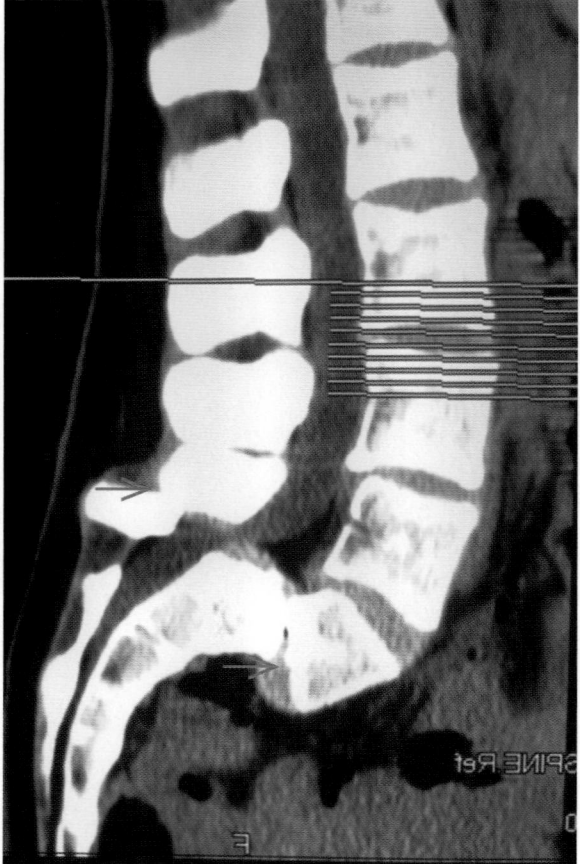

● **Fig. 8.7** Lateral magnetic resonance imaging (MRI) scan of lumbar spine showing uncorrected spondylolisthesis with marked anterior displacement of L5 on S1 (arrows). Epidural block at L2–3 was satisfactory.

AP view (Fig. 8.8c) reveals the limited volume of contrast extending down to T10/11 on the left (arrowed), while the lateral aspect (Fig. 8.8d) shows contrast up to T5 (arrowed).

The patient made a perfect recovery, and was sailing her windsurfer 2 weeks postpartum.

CASE HISTORY 8.6:
SATISFACTORY BLOCK FOLLOWING SPINAL FIXATION

A 35-year-old with a breech presentation was scheduled for elective caesarean section. She suffered marked scoliosis in adolescence and underwent Harrington rod fixation at the age of 15 years. Two years previously, in her first labour, epidural catheterization at L3–4 had been straightforward, but the resulting block was

predominantly right-sided and was not corrected despite additional doses of local anaesthetic and partial catheter withdrawal.

When reviewed, with her radiographs, in the third trimester, she reported occasional lower back pains during the pregnancy, which improved with physiotherapy. The extensive paramedian surgical scarring on the back was noted. Prior to surgery, midline epidural puncture was undertaken at L2–3, just below the end of the surgical scar, and 5 cm of a terminal eye catheter (Arrow) inserted into the epidural space, at the third attempt. Following 20 mL ropivacaine 0.875% a totally right-sided block to T4 developed over 20 min. After a further 15 mL over the next 25 min, a left-sided block had appeared, but only to T10. The patient was informed that the block was not entirely satisfactory, but she elected for surgery to commence, and was comfortable apart from some brief, sharp, left-sided upper abdominal pain on peritoneal mobilization. An epidurogram was performed the following day.

Epiduroram findings; scoliosis, predominantly unilateral block

On fluoroscopic screening, the epidural catheter was seen to be partially obscured by the tip of the lower rod (Fig. 8.9a) at L2–3, with the catheter well to the right of the midline. The initial flow of contrast was entirely right-sided, following the inside of the curve, as expected, with only minimal spread across the midline. The enlarged AP epidurogram following 10 mL of contrast (Fig. 8.9b) reveals the predominantly unilateral contrast spread from L1 to L5 (blue arrows) with marked right foraminal spill at most levels (red arrows), and sparse spread of contrast on the left. In the lateral view (Fig. 8.9c), the lumbar spine appeared very straight, with loss of the normal lumbar lordosis and contrast fairly uniformly spread across the lumbar epidural space.

CASE HISTORY 8.7:
POOR SACRAL BLOCK

A 78-year-old patient presented for vaginal hysterectomy, and gave a history of laminectomy and spinal fusion for chronic disc disease. She had no current back symptoms. Epidural puncture was performed uneventfully at the closest interspace to the cephalad end of the laminectomy scar, T12–L1, and 3 cm of a terminal eye 19 gauge catheter (Arrow) inserted into the epidural space. Following the injection of 15 mL lidocaine 1.5% in the sitting position, the block extended up to T8 bilaterally, but with only patchy sacral numbness to pinprick. There was perineal discomfort at the start

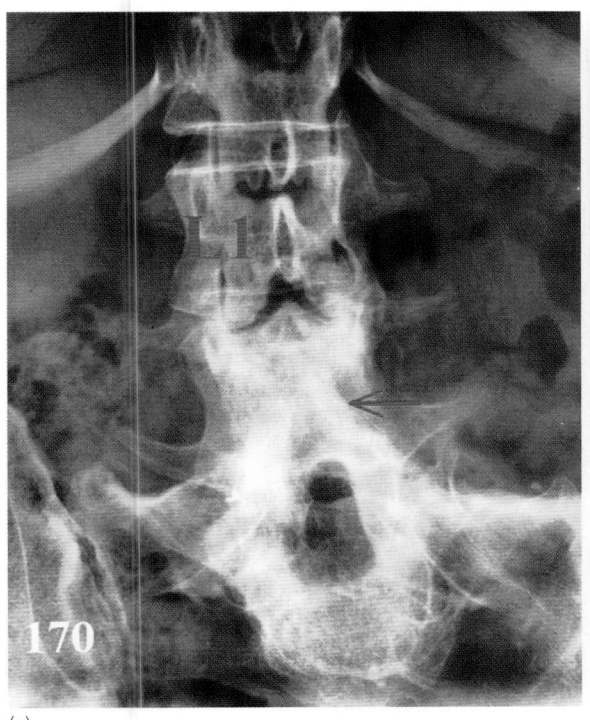

(a)

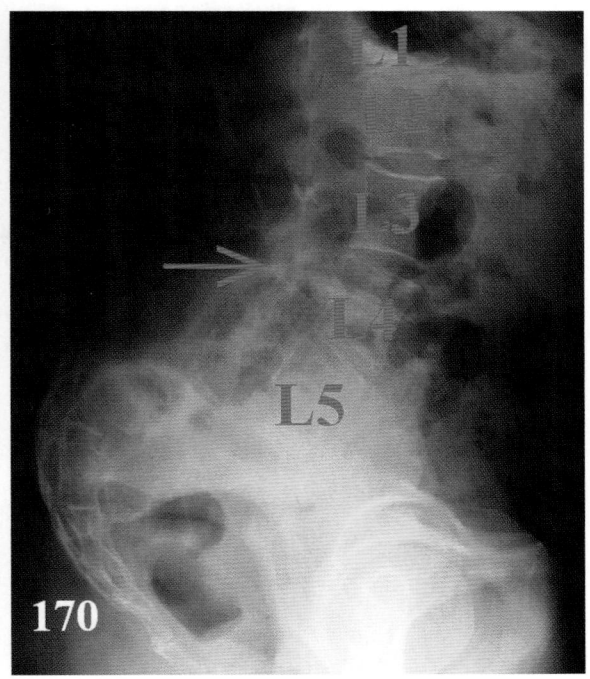

(b)

● **Fig. 8.8**
(a) Anteroposterior (AP)
radiograph following
spinal fusion for L5–S1
spondylolisthesis. Below
L1, vertebral anatomy
is grossly distorted,
with bone grafts and
new bone formation
(arrowed). (b) Lateral
radiograph following
spinal fusion for L5–S1
spondylolisthesis. Marked
lumbar lordosis and
acute sacral angulation
are evident, in addition
to the fusion of L4 to S1,
with bone grafts and new
bone formation (arrowed).
(c) An AP epidurogram
following 6 mL of contrast.
The catheter tip was seen
at the T9–10 interspace,
with contrast extending
down to T10–11 on the
left (arrowed). (d) Lateral
epidurogram following
6 mL of contrast. Contrast
spread is fairly uniform
between T5 and T11.

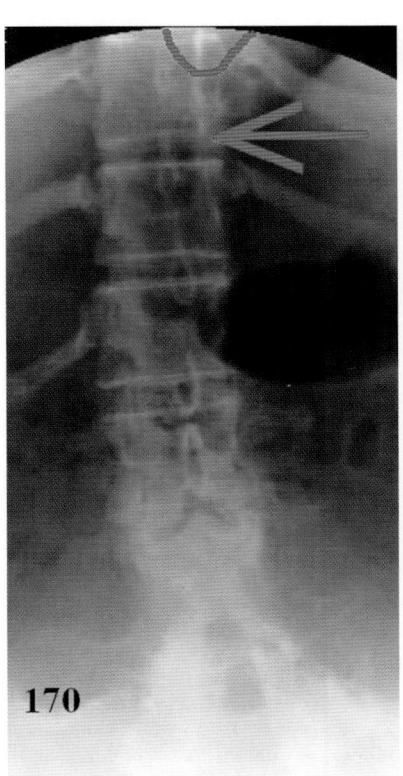

(c)

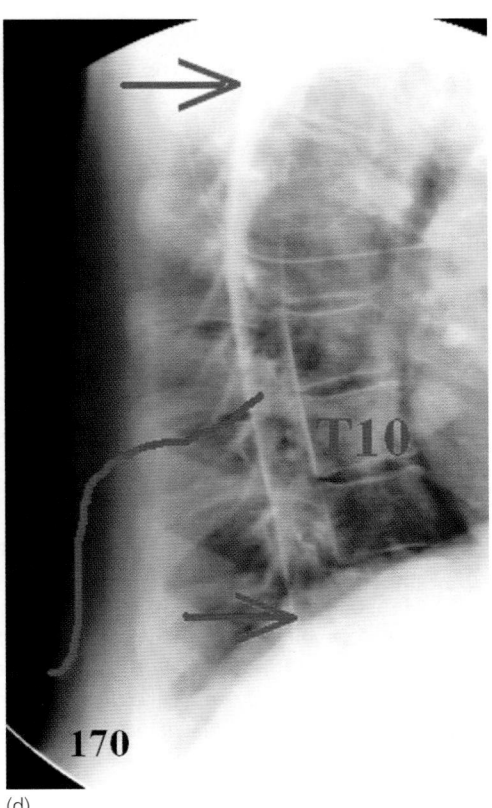

(d)

● **Fig. 8.9**
(a) Anteroposterior (AP) radiograph showing scoliosis and Harrington rods, with the lumbar curve convex to the left, and the catheter tip at L2–3, to the right of the midline. (b) An AP epidurogram (magnified) showing predominantly right-sided distribution of contrast, from L1 to L5 (blue arrows), with marked right transforaminal spill (red arrows).

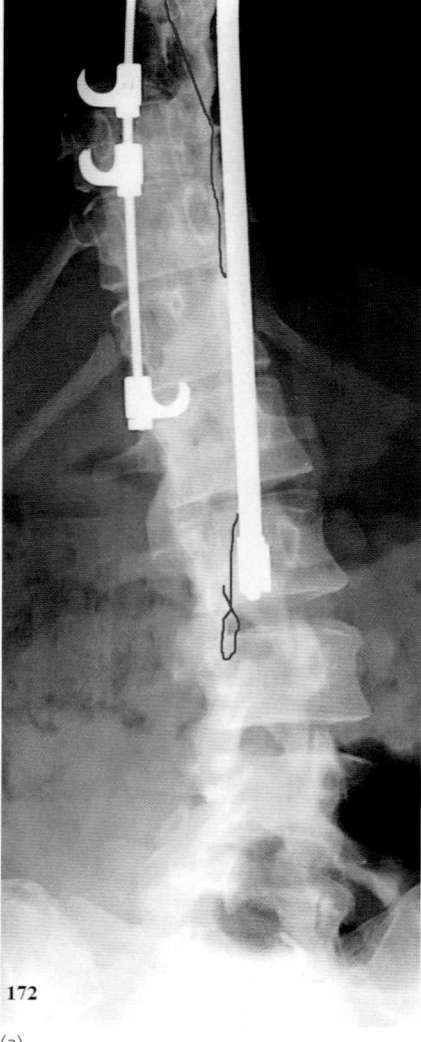

(a)

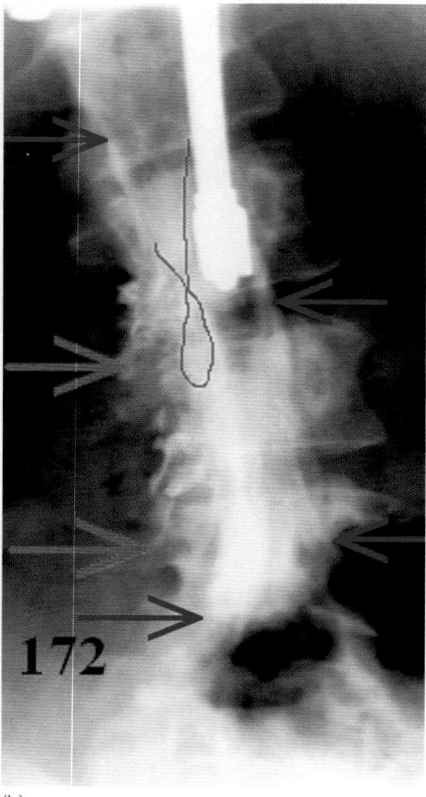

(b)

of surgery, but this was relieved by local anaesthetic infiltration.

Epidurogram findings: **restricted lumbar contrast spread**

On fluoroscopic screening there was marked degenerative bone disease with laminectomies at L3, L4 and L5, and screw fixation of L4 and L5 (Fig. 8.10a). The radio-opaque catheter was visible at T12, with its tip in the midline, pointing cephalad. The injection of 13 mL of contrast over 30 s appeared as a dense collection between T12 and L2 showing considerable lumbar foraminal spill. Contrast would not flow below L2, despite the injection of a further 7 mL of contrast. The AP epidurogram (Fig. 8.10a) revealed the final picture, with the upper level

of contrast at T4 (above upper arrow) and the lower end at L2, with a fairly sharp cut-off point (lower arrow). In the lateral radiograph (Fig. 8.10b) the epidural contrast flow again appears to be abruptly obstructed below L2, probably to be replaced by a dense mass of fibrous tissue (lower arrow). Above this, there is fairly satisfactory and uniform contrast flow across the epidural space, although a few small filling defects are present. Presumably, the presence of surgical adhesions impeded the caudal spread of both the epidural local anaesthetic and the subsequent contrast.

These three example Case Histories illustrate some of the difficulties that may arise in the management of epidural blocks in patients with spinal pathology and surgical

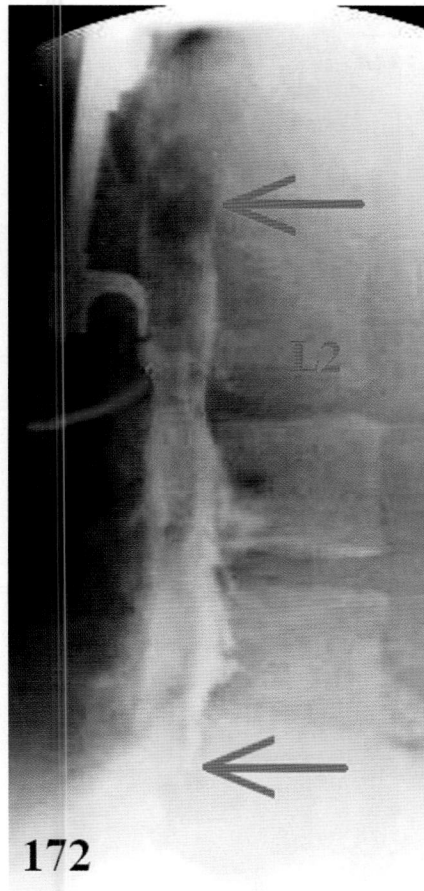

172

(c)

● **Fig. 8.9** (Continued) (c) Lateral epidurogram revealing the lower end of a Harrington rod with a loss of lumbar lordosis and contrast flowing fairly uniformly across (the right side of) the epidural space from L1 to L5.

correction. These difficulties can usually be overcome by increasing the volume of local anaesthetic, sometimes with the simultaneous use of two epidural catheters at adjacent interspaces,[3] but a perfect block cannot always be expected.

8.4 Congenital block vertebrae

FLUID ASPIRATION THROUGH A LUMBAR EPIDURAL CATHETER

A 28-year-old patient with a history of chronic mild backache underwent abdominal hysterectomy under satisfactory epidural block at L3–4. The initial 20 mL dose

of local anaesthetic was given incrementally through the Tuohy needle. The only unusual feature during the course of block insertion was the ability to aspirate the local anaesthetic freely after each 5 mL dose. Similarly, 3–5 mL of clear fluid could be aspirated through the epidural catheter (three lateral eyes, Portex) for up to 1 h after each of three 10 mL top-up doses for postoperative analgesia, which proved effective. On each occasion the fluid was tested to exclude the presence of cerebrospinal fluid (CSF). As the patient was allergic to iodine no contrast was injected.

Radiographic findings: congenital block vertebrae
The AP and lateral views (Fig. 8.11) show congenital block vertebrae, with fusion of T12/L1 and L2/3, and a wide intervertebral space between the bodies of L3/4 and L4/L5. There is a mild scoliosis, and the vertebral canal is of larger diameter than usual (arrowed).

Block vertebrae are a fairly frequent finding in routine radiographs and are thought to result from a developmental failure of segmentation.[9] A wider epidural space than usual may have allowed a large pool of epidural local anaesthetic to accumulate, from which aspiration was possible, initially through the Tuohy needle, and later through the catheter. This ability to aspirate was a rare occurrence, with an incidence of approximately 1 in 500 blocks in our hands, and caused concern that dural puncture may have occurred.

8.5 Spina bifida occulta

As spina bifida occulta (SBO) is commonly noted on routine radiological examination of the lumbosacral spine, it was inevitable that we would detect many examples in our series of 181 cases (three patients did not have epidurograms). Another four parturients with SBO were referred to us for antepartum assessment, but did not require regional anaesthesia. We have attempted to assess the relevance of this anomaly to epidural block function, particularly in parturients.

The condition of spina bifida occulta is only rarely mentioned in anaesthesia textbooks, and slightly more commonly in journal articles, in which the published work can sometimes be misleading. For example, in 1988, after discussing a patient with minor radiological changes typical of SBO, the authors conclude erroneously that 'Attempted epidural puncture at the level of the lesion will almost certainly result in a dural tap.[10] A case report from 1996 warns against epidural block in patients with spina bifida.[11] This condition clearly needs some clarification and an explanation of the various categories follows.

● **Fig. 8.10**
(a) Anteroposterior (AP) epidurogram revealing laminectomies at L3, L4 and L5 with screw fixation at L4–5. The body of contrast extends from T8 to an abrupt cut-off at L2 (lower arrow) and is a little fragmented. The only significant foraminal spill is at L1 and L2. (b) Lateral epidurogram post-laminectomy. The epidural space appears disrupted below L2 (lower arrow), with an irregular edge to the contrast, suggesting a fibrous reaction.

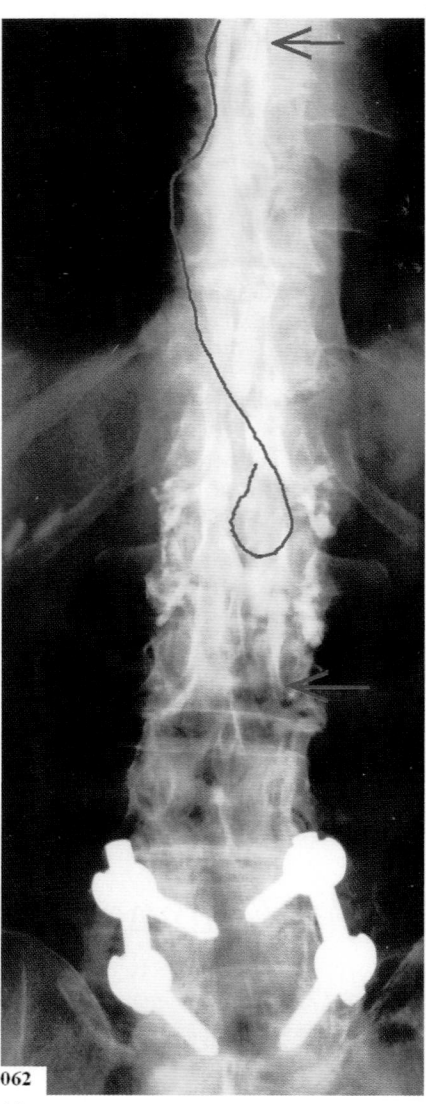

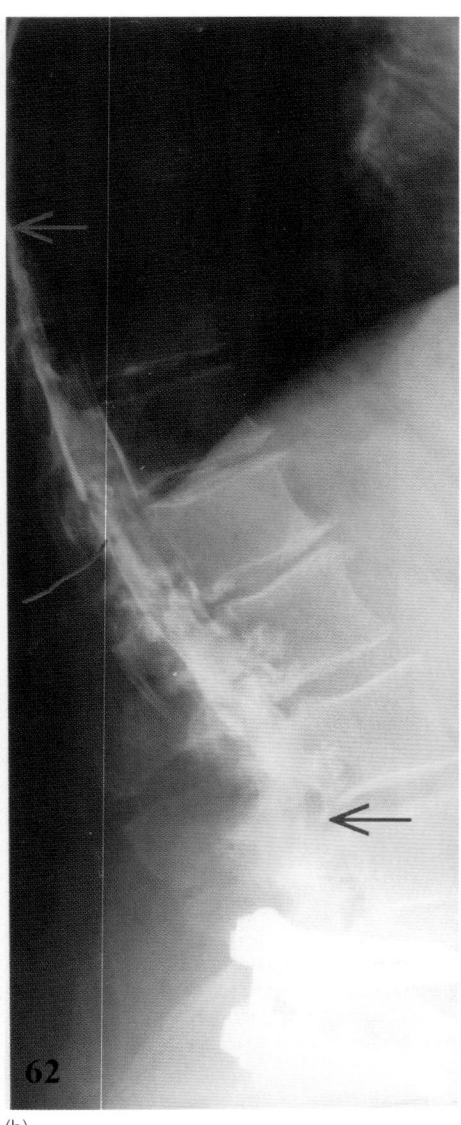

(a)

(b)

8.5.1 **Spinal dysraphism**

This is a term that describes all defects associated with a failure of closure of the posterior neural arch. There is some confusion in the literature as to the precise classification of these defects[12] but division into three groups may be helpful.

8.5.1.1 Spina bifida cystica

The most severely affected individuals display spina bifida cystica (or aperta), which involves complex bony abnormalities with cystic protrusion of neural elements in the form of a meningocele or myelomeningocele. In the

past, these defects were rarely encountered in pregnant women, but with increased life expectancy and quality of life, this has changed and many successful blocks have been reported.[13]

8.5.1.2 Spina bifida occulta

This is an extremely common condition, being present as a radiological finding in 5–20% of individuals in Australasia, and 18–34% of the population of the USA.[14] It comprises incomplete formation of a single lamina, or occasionally two adjacent laminae, most commonly in the lumbosacral region, without any other abnormalities. The bony defect is

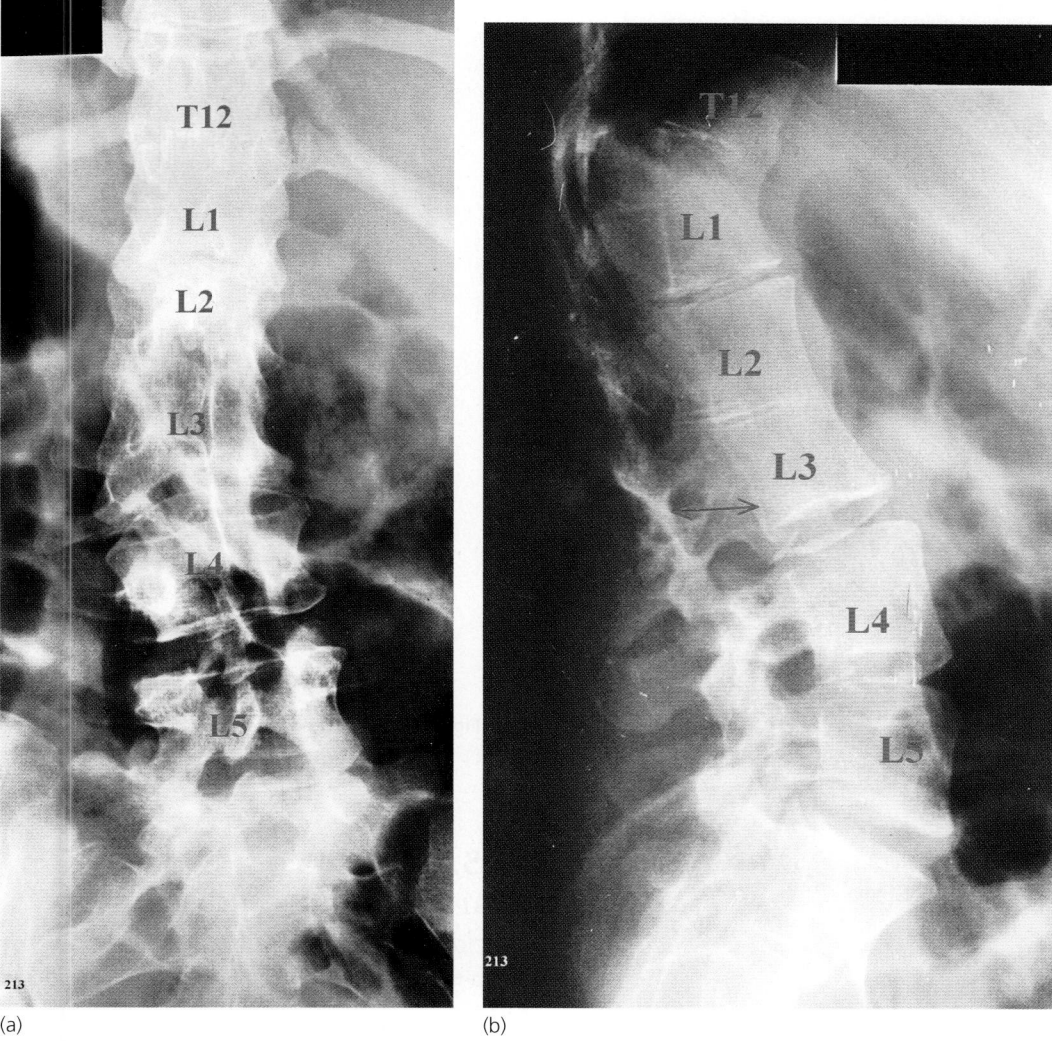

(a)   (b)

● **Fig. 8.11** (a) Anteroposterior (AP) radiograph of congenital lumbar block vertebrae. (b) Lateral radiograph of congenital lumbar block vertebrae, with relatively wide vertebral canal (arrowed).

not thought to be clinically significant and epidural or spinal anaesthesia may be safely undertaken. The radiological appearance is usually an incidental finding (Figs 8.12 and 8.13, both associated with satisfactory blocks), and many radiologists do not consider it worthwhile to include it in their routine reports.

8.5.1.3 Occult spinal dysraphism

There is a third, intermediate group where the bony defect is associated with spinal abnormalities of varying degrees of severity.[12] These include intraspinal lipomas, dermal sinus tracts, dermoid cysts, fibrous bands and diastematomyelia (congenital splitting of the cord, by a bony, fibrous or cartilaginous spur). These patients may have no neurological symptoms, or only minor lower limb motor or sensory defects, with or without bladder dysfunction. A tethered cord is one that extends below the L2–3 interspace and is found in many of these patients, who often display cutaneous manifestations overlying the bony anomaly such as a tuft of hair, a dimple, a sinus, or port wine stain or other haemangioma or naevus. Patients with these signs in the thoracolumbar area, or neurological symptoms, or radiological evidence of failure of fusion of more than a single spinal lamina, should have tethering of the cord

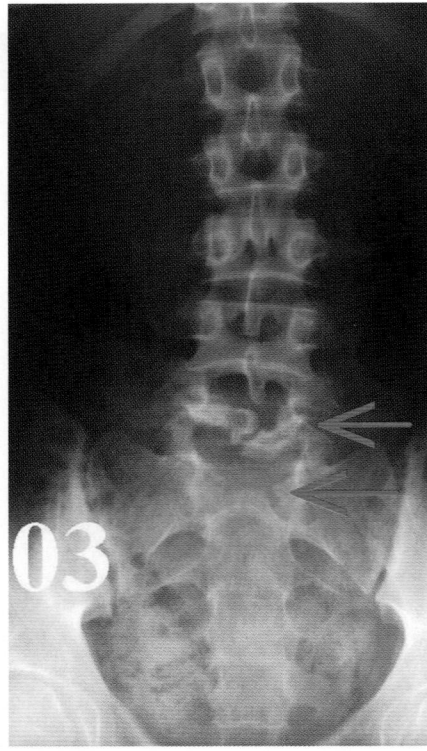

Fig. 8.12 Anteroposterior (AP) radiograph of L5 and S1 spina bifida (arrowed). Epidural block was satisfactory.

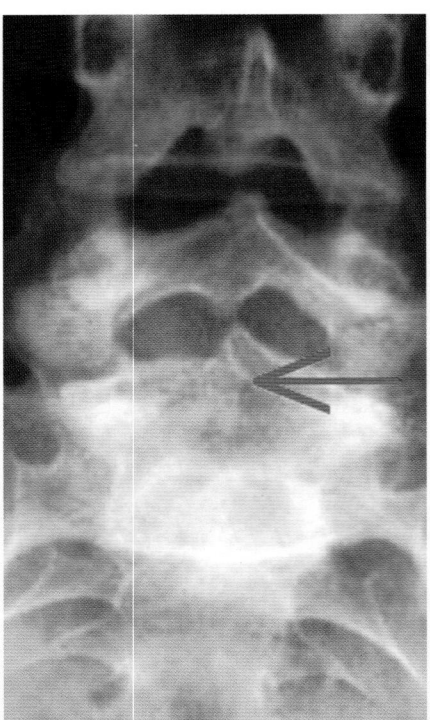

Fig. 8.13 Anteroposterior (AP) radiograph of S1 spina bifida (arrowed). Epidural block was satisfactory.

excluded by magnetic resonance imaging (MRI) examination before epidural or spinal anaesthesia. We have detected two patients with a dermal sinus tract and two other patients with unusually prominent midline 'moles' (naevi); all in association with spina bifida occulta.

One parturient was investigated for persistent severe lower backache in early pregnancy and displayed congenital lumbar hemivertebrae, another reasonably common vertebral anomaly, on her radiographs, in addition to spina bifida at S1 (Fig. 8.14, arrowed). Regional block was not requested for delivery.

8.5.2 Results of this study

Of our 181 cases, there was evidence of spinal dysraphism in 22, with two individuals presenting twice in consecutive pregnancies, so that 20 individual patients were studied and the overall incidence of this deformity was 12.2%. Only 4 of the 20 patients were aware of the condition before initial epidural block and, helpfully, they had brought their radiographs to a consultation with an anaesthetist before hospital admission. Eighteen individuals had SBO and two had occult spinal dysraphism with a dermal sinus tract.

8.5.2.1 Spina bifida occulta in parturients

Incidence of spina bifida occulta

Eighteen cases of SBO occurred in our series of 146 parturients (12.3%) and these are discussed first (Fig. 8.15). The other four cases were discovered in gynaecological surgery patients. In three cases the epidural block was entirely satisfactory, in six the block was complicated and in another nine it was unsatisfactory, at least initially. These results are hardly surprising as the primary aim of our study was to investigate complicated or unsatisfactory blocks.

Complicated blocks with spina bifida occulta (Fig. 8.15)

Reviewing the six parturients with complicated blocks in the presence of SBO, five cases involved intradural injection and the other a recurring high block (Fig. 8.15).

Intradural injection and spina bifida occulta

In the group of 10 patients with intradural injection (see Chapter 5, section 5.2.2, p.50) all had patchy blocks of slow onset, which eventually responded to repeated doses of local anaesthetic, occasionally with extensive blocks resulting.

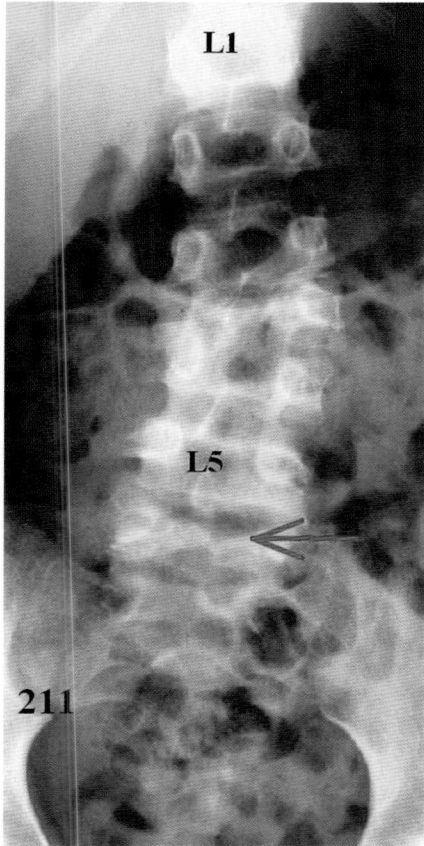

Fig. 8.14 Anteroposterior (AP) radiograph showing congenital lumbar hemivertebrae and spina bifida at S1 (arrowed). No regional block required.

The radiographs of five revealed the presence of intradural injection together with mild defects of fusion of the S1 lamina. Two examples are shown (Figs 8.16 and 8.17). The numbers are too small and the patient sampling too selective for valid statistical analysis, and more data are required, but it is interesting to speculate as to whether there could be any connection between the presence of SBO and the resulting intradural injection. We do not know why intradural injection occurs. It has been reported after attempted epidural block by highly experienced anaesthetists, following apparently routine needle and catheter insertion.[15] It is possible, in the patient with SBO, that there is a related congenital defect of the ligamentum flavum or dura, or both, which predisposes that individual to unwitting entry of the needle or catheter into the intradural space, but this is highly speculative and more information is being sought.

Recurring high epidural block and SBO

This patient with a recurring high block developed an extensive neuraxial block prior to caesarean section, with numbness up to C6 and trigeminal nerve involvement following a 20 mL dose of ropivacaine 1.0%. A similar high block had developed during labour 2 years previously

Occult spinal dysraphism
in parturients = 18 cases

Complicated = 6   Satisfactory = 3   Failed = 9

Intradural = 5
High epidural = 1
(pars defect)

Unilateral (patchy) = 7
Missed segment = 1
Intravascular = 1

Fig. 8.15 Outcome of epidural blocks in 18 parturients with spinal dysraphism.

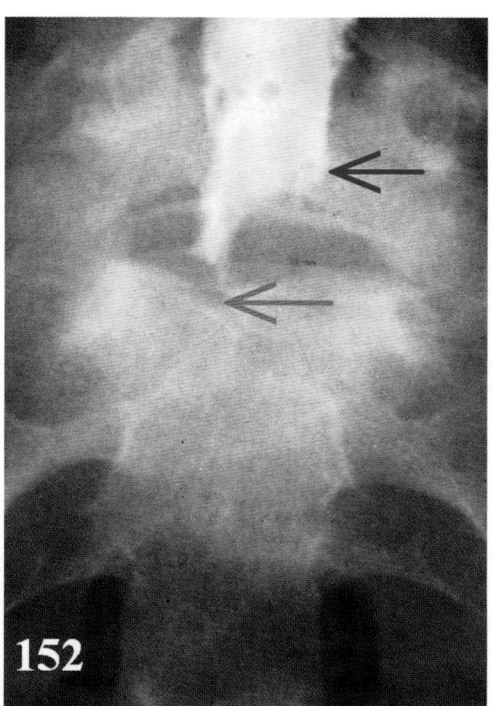

Fig. 8.16 Anteroposterior (AP) epidurogram (magnified) showing spina bifida occulta at S1 (red arrow), in the presence of the caudal end of a mass of intradural contrast (blue arrow). Same patient as in Fig. 5.14b, p.61.

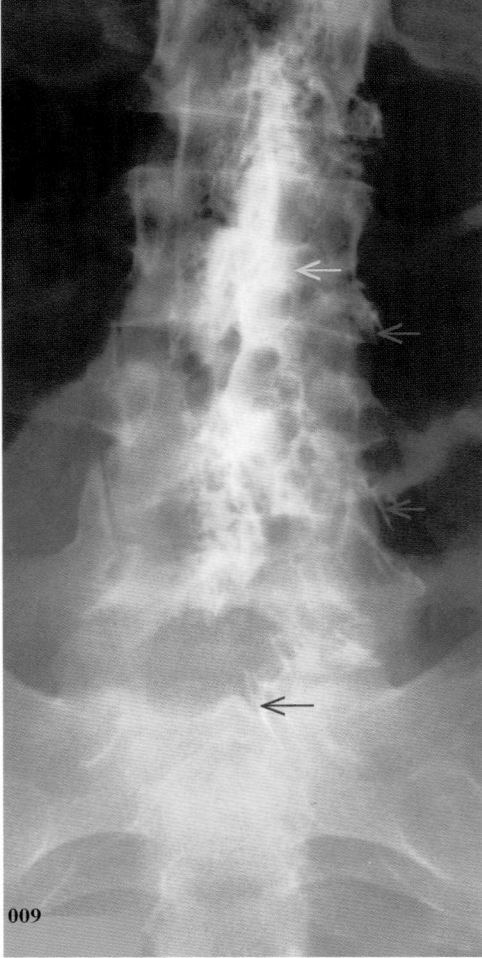

● **Fig. 8.17** Anteroposterior (AP) epidurogram showing spina bifida occulta at S1(red arrow), with transforaminal spill of epidural contrast (blue arrows) and dense intradural contrast (yellow arrow).

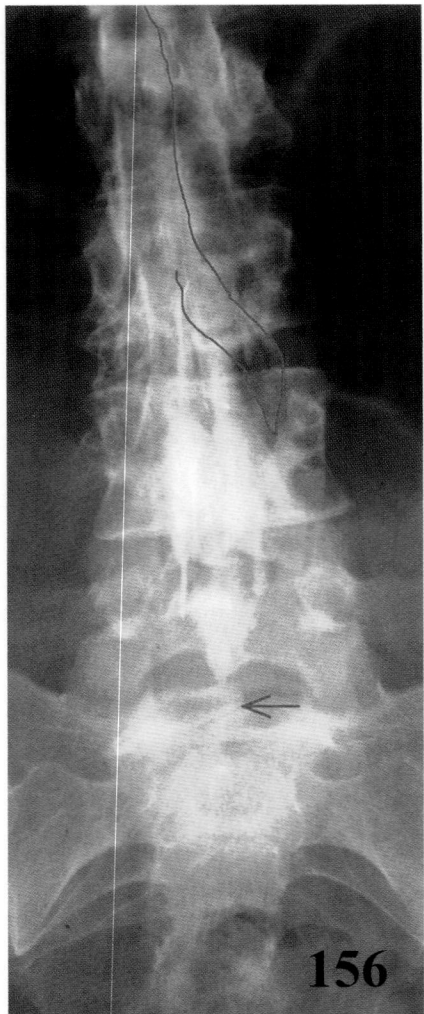

● **Fig. 8.18** Anteroposterior (AP) epidurogram of lumbar spine showing mild scoliosis with spina bifida occulta at S1 (arrowed), and fairly typical epidural contrast spread following a high block.

following 15 mL bupivacaine 0.125%. Epidurogram post-caesarean revealed a fairly typical contrast spread (Fig. 8.18) from T11 to L4, with spina bifida at S1. The finding of SBO appeared to be entirely coincidental.

Unsatisfactory blocks and spina bifida occulta (Fig. 8.15)

There were nine unsatisfactory blocks in the 18 obstetric cases with SBO, of whom seven had unilateral or patchy blocks in labour, associated with a demonstrated midline septum in four (Fig. 8.15). Six of these cases had required epidural catheter replacement (two examples are Figs 8.19 and 8.20) and the seventh responded to partial catheter withdrawal.

One of the six patients requiring catheter replacement had a coexisting pars interarticularis defect (see below). The eighth case of unsatisfactory block presented with severe localized lower abdominal pain at caesarean section due to an apparent 'missed segment' at T10–T11. The AP epidurogram showed the abrupt cut-off of epidural contrast at L1 on the same side (Fig. 8.21, upper arrow) and SBO at S1 (lower arrow).

The final (ninth) case involved partial intravenous injection through the epidural catheter, with signs of local anaesthetic toxicity. No obvious connection between any of these unsatisfactory blocks and SBO was apparent.

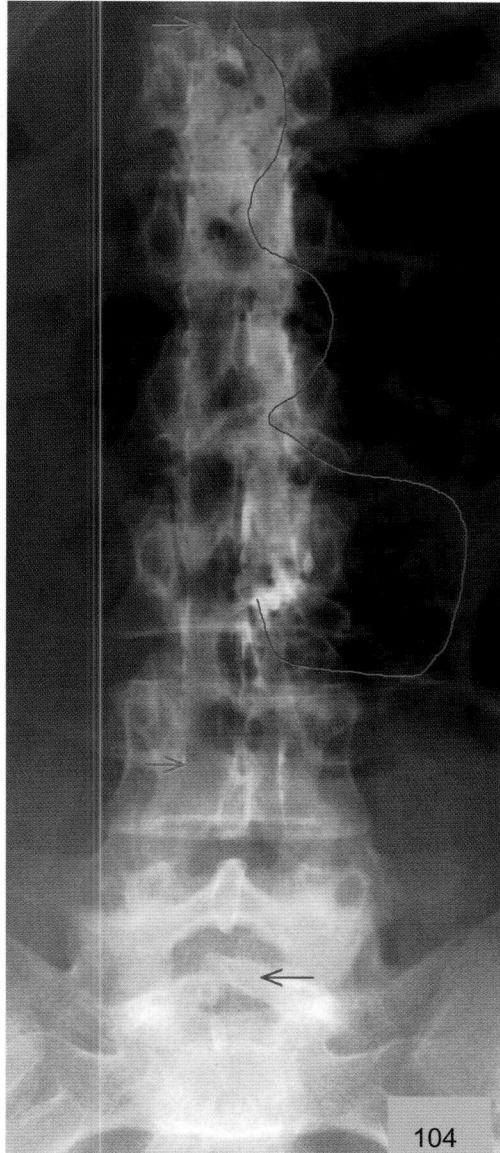

Fig. 8.19 Anteroposterior (AP) epidurogram showing spina bifida occulta at S1 (lower arrow), associated with predominantly left-sided contrast (upper arrows) following unilateral block, almost certainly caused by a midline septum.

8.5.2.2 Spina bifida occulta and pars interarticularis defect

There appears to be a close relationship between SBO and other bony vertebral lesions such as pars interarticularis defects and spondylolisthesis,[8] as well as hemivertebrae, as already seen. Any possible role for these abnormalities in the development of unsatisfactory blocks is unknown.

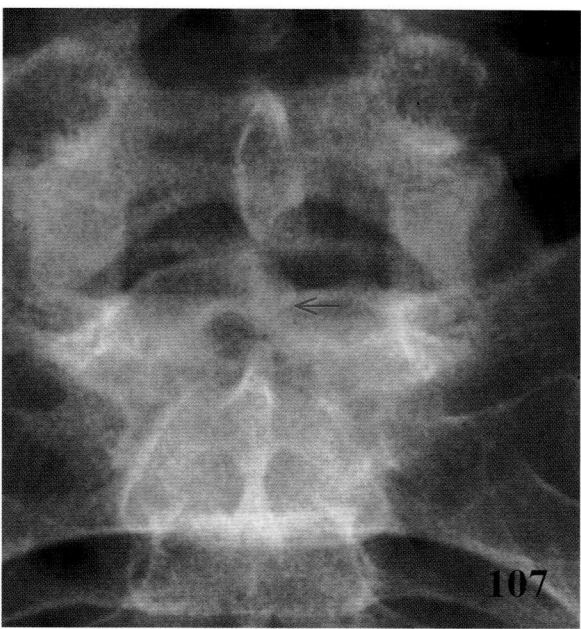

Fig. 8.20 Anteroposterior (AP) radiograph (magnified) of lumbosacral junction showing spina bifida occulta at S1 (arrowed), following a persistent predominantly left unilateral block.

CASE HISTORY 8.9:
RECURRING UNSATISFACTORY BLOCK WITH 2 BONY DEFECTS

A 35-year-old patient in her first labour requested an epidural block. The anaesthetist noted an unusual slightly raised mole in the midline over the body of L4, in the absence of any other such lesions on the back. There was no history of chronic backache or spina bifida occulta. Epidural puncture at L3–4 required two attempts before a terminal eye catheter (Arrow) was inserted 4 cm into the epidural space. The block was satisfactory for 7 h, but then the patient complained of persistent severe lower abdominal and perineal pain despite repeated top-up doses of ropivacaine 0.2%. The block was found on pinprick testing to extend up to T8, but to spare the lumbosacral roots.

The epidural insertion site was inspected and the catheter was found to have been extruded by 4 cm under intact fixation, presumably as a result of excessive pressure within the epidural space. There had been considerable backflow through the Tuohy needle on initial injection and the continuous infusion pump had occluded on several occasions. A second catheter at L2–3 provided successful analgesia for labour and delivery.

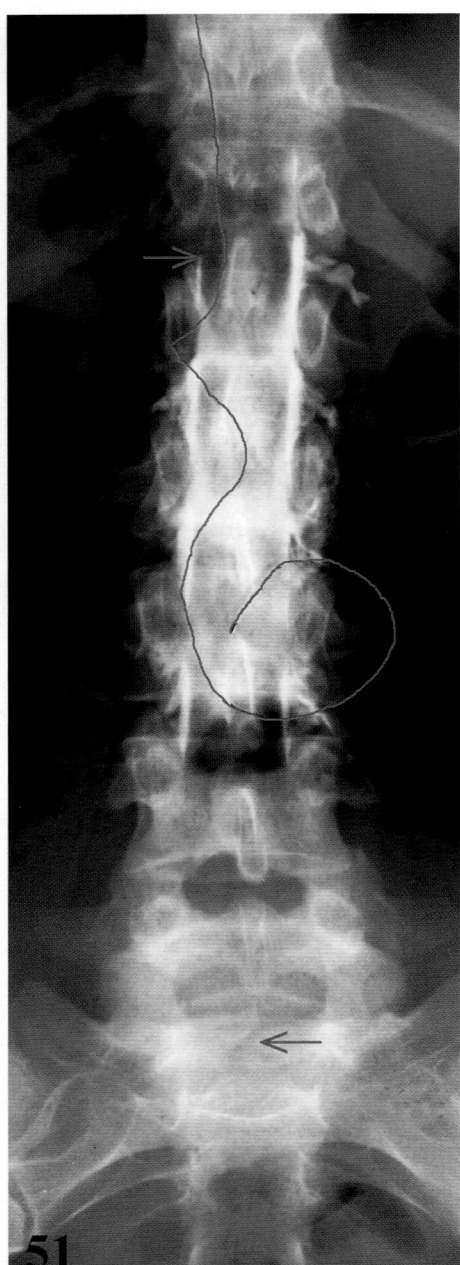

● **Fig. 8.21** Anteroposterior (AP) epidurogram showing spina bifida occulta at S1 (lower arrow), with restricted spread of epidural contrast from T12 to L4, following a 'missed segment block' with persistent right sided T10–11 abdominal pain during labour. The spread of contrast is abruptly cut off at L1 on the right (upper arrow).

Radiographic findings: restricted contrast spread, spina bifida occulta, pars defect

An epidurogram on the following day using 12 mL of contrast revealed a restricted spread of epidural contrast from T10 to L3, with minimal lower lumbar and sacral flow (Fig. 8.22a, arrowed). The radiologist reported 'sclerosis in the region of the pars interarticularis at the L5 level (blue arrows), suggesting pars interarticularis defect' in addition to spina bifida occulta at S1 (lower red arrow). A magnified view is seen in Fig. 8.22b, although an oblique view may be the preferred image to detect a pars defect.

Pars interarticularis defects (or simply 'pars defects')[8] are well known to orthopaedic surgeons and sports medicine specialists, and may occur in up to 5% of the population. The defect, also known as 'spondylolysis' refers to an interruption of the vertebral arch at the bony bridge that holds together the superior and inferior articular processes that form the facet joints. This failure of fusion of the pars may be either a congenital defect or post-traumatic. The defect may be unilateral or bilateral, when it may be associated with spondylolisthesis. In our patient the defect was bilateral, and was not particularly obvious in our lateral radiographs. Up to 30% of patients with a pars defect also demonstrate SBO.

Any possible role played by spina bifida occulta and a coexisting pars defect in the development of this patient's failed epidural block remains a matter of conjecture, as does the presence of the overlaying naevus.

8.5.2.3 Spina bifida occulta and skin lesions

Another of the parturients was noted to have an unusual prominent raised midline mole over the upper body of L2, with another smaller mole nearby (Fig. 8.23a). The pigmented naevi in the absence of other similar lesions raised a vague suspicion of the presence of spinal dysraphism, even though the lesions were well away from the usual L5 and S1 sites for spina bifida. Epidural block for labour was inserted at L3–4, with some difficulty, but after four attempts proved entirely satisfactory. Radiography the following day revealed a mild scoliosis and SBO with a failure of fusion at S1 (Fig. 8.23b), and satisfactory contrast spread. In this case, once again, the presence of the unusual mole appeared to be entirely coincidental and not representative of occult spinal dysraphism, although this cannot be absolutely excluded without computed tomography (CT) or MRI scan.

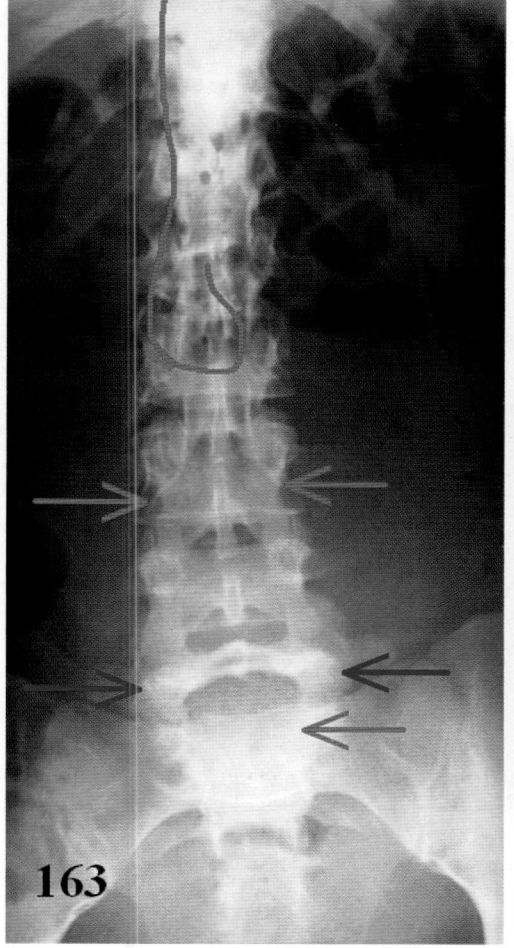
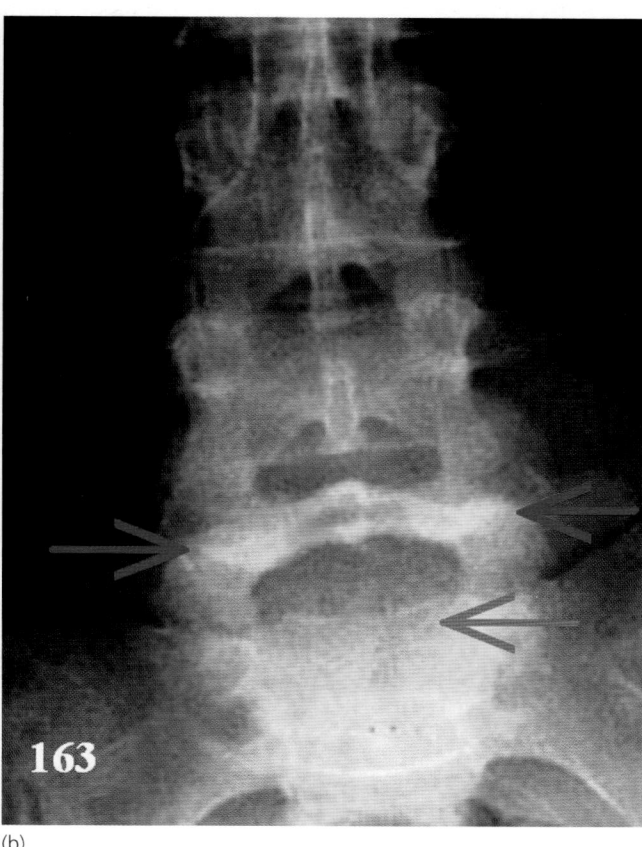

(a)   (b)

● **Fig. 8.22** (a) Anteroposterior (AP) epidurogram, showing pars interarticularis defects at L5 (blue arrows) and spina bifida occulta at S1 (lower red arrow), with a restricted caudal spread of epidural contrast to L3 only (upper arrows) following a poor block of sacral nerve roots. (b) An AP epidurogram providing a close-up view of pars interarticularis defects at L5 (blue arrows) and spina bifida occulta at S1 (red arrow).

8.5.2.4 Results in non-obstetric patients with spina bifida occulta

Epidurograms were undertaken on 32 gynaecological patients, of whom four were found to have SBO. In one, the block had been satisfactory, in another there was a failure to locate the epidural space and the contrast was located in the paravertebral space (Fig. 6.7a, p.80), while in the other two, the block was found to be unilateral in one and too

high in the other. No conclusions could be reached as to causation.

8.5.3 Occult spinal dysraphism

Only two of the 22 cases of spinal dysraphism fell into this category, with both patients having a dermal sinus tract. This congenital defect results from a failure of separation

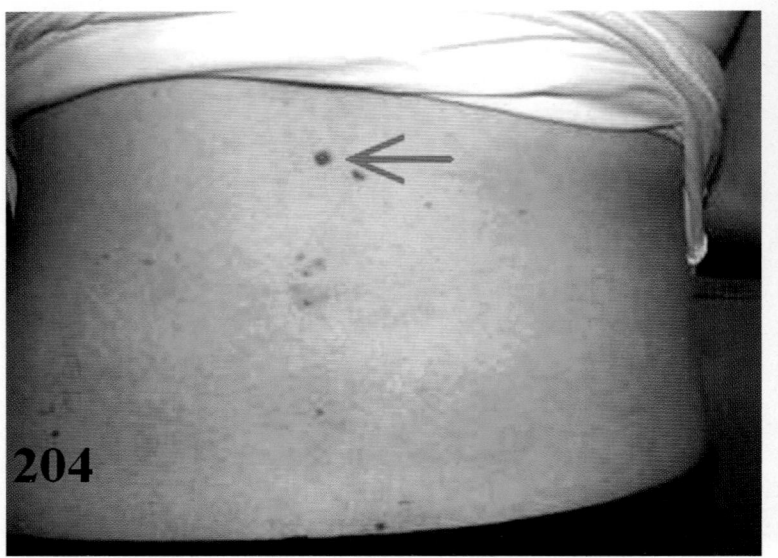

(a)

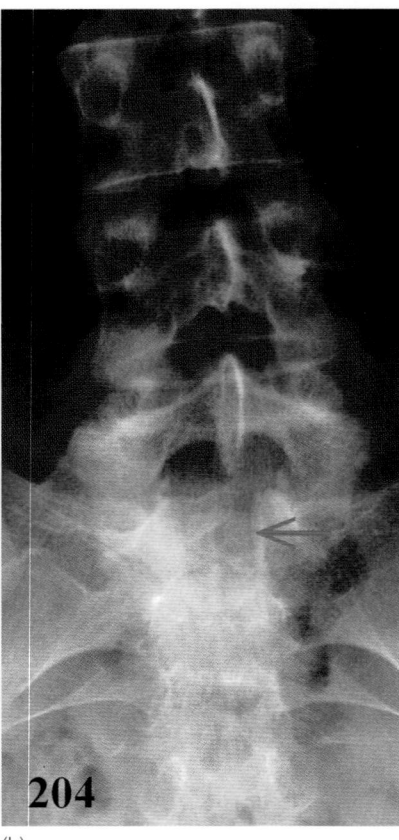

(b)

● **Fig. 8.23** (a) View of patient's back with prominent midline mole at L2 (arrowed), and multiple puncture marks at L3–4. (b) Anteroposterior (AP) radiograph demonstrating spina bifida at S1, in the same patient.

of neuronal from epithelial ectoderm. This may coexist with other midline fusion defects, with or without a tethered cord. The sinus may represent the opening of a blind-ending duct, as in our first case, or may extend into the spinal canal, as in our second case.

CASE HISTORY 8.10:
SPINA BIFIDA WITH DERMAL SINUS

A 37-year-old patient had a small dermal sinus tract at the level of her coccyx (Fig. 8.24a) and SBO at S1/2 (Fig. 8.24b), with a wide 'V-shaped' fusion defect in the posterior sacrum. This patient had epidural blocks inserted in all of her four labours. All four blocks were predominantly unilateral on the left, with the catheters having to be resited on two occasions, with

little improvement in block quality. Unfortunately, no epidurograms were undertaken.

CASE HISTORY 8.11:
SPINA BIFIDA WITH DERMAL SINUS

A 40-year-old patient from a remote country town presented for abdominal hysterectomy, without any previous medical or surgical history. Since childhood, she had been aware of a 'small lump' over her lumbar spine, which occasionally discharged 'a little watery fluid', but otherwise did not trouble her, and medical advice had not been sought. On examination of her back, a large dimple was discovered in the midline at L4–5 (Fig. 8.25a), with an adjacent soft reddish cystic mass, approximately 5 mm in diameter, topped by a punctum (Fig. 8.25b).

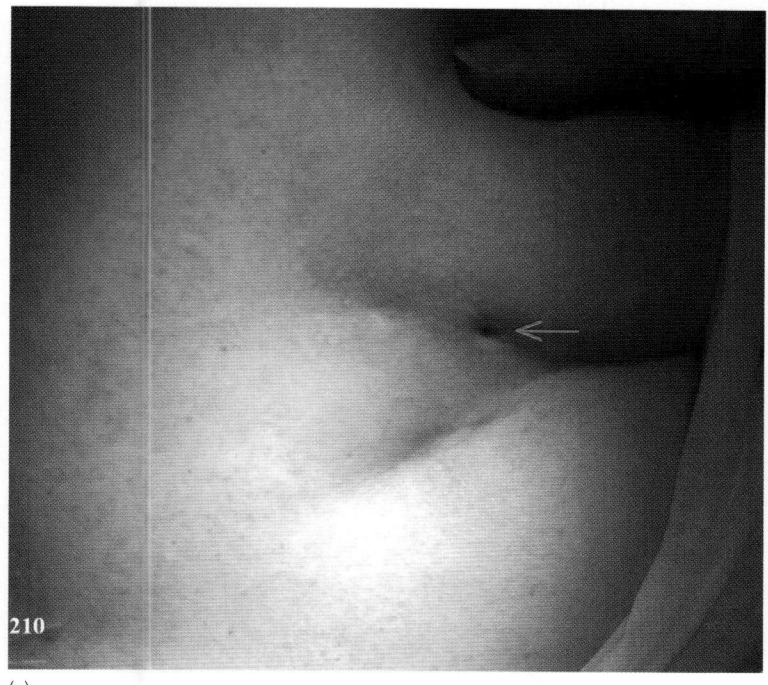

(a)

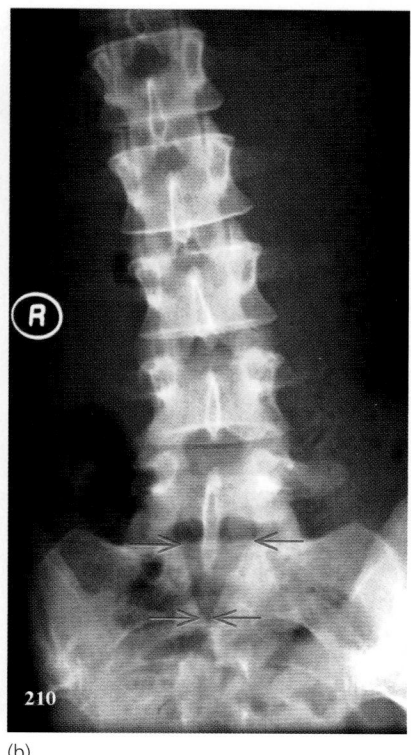

(b)

Fig. 8.24 (a) Photograph of lower back and buttocks with the patient in the left lateral position, showing the opening of a dermal sinus tract on the right side of the coccyx (arrowed). This is associated with six unsatisfactory epidural blocks in four labours and spina bifida occulta at S1/S2. (b) Anteroposterior (AP) radiograph in same patient showing spina bifida in the form of a V-shaped defect (arrowed), resulting from failure of fusion of the posterior elements of S1 and S2.

No fluid could be expressed on the exertion of gentle pressure.

As she also suffered micrognathism, with extremely limited mouth opening, endotracheal intubation was expected to be difficult, if not impossible, and regional anaesthesia was planned for surgery with the patient's consent.

Radiographic findings: spina bifida S1

Anteroposterior radiography of the thoracolumbar spine revealed an asymmetrical failure of fusion of the S1 laminae, with associated distortion at L5 (Fig. 8.25c). Epidural block at L2–3 was undertaken successfully, and there were no complications. This case occurred many years ago, prior to the introduction of CT or MRI scans, which would be advisable today as part of any preoperative assessment.

8.5.4 Summary of findings on spina bifida occulta

There have been many previous attempts to link the presence of SBO to a clinically significant problem, such as lower urinary tract dysfunction[16] or chronic back pain,[17] but with only limited success. With regard to the efficiency of epidural block in the presence of SBO the results are inconclusive at this stage, but the finding of several cases of unilateral block or intradural injection co-existing with SBO is interesting and further investigation is required.

The presence of an isolated raised pigmented lesion in the midline of the lumbosacral area will almost certainly be coincidental on most occasions, but might possibly be an indication of an underlying spina bifida occulta at the same or a different vertebral level, but more data are also required on this aspect.

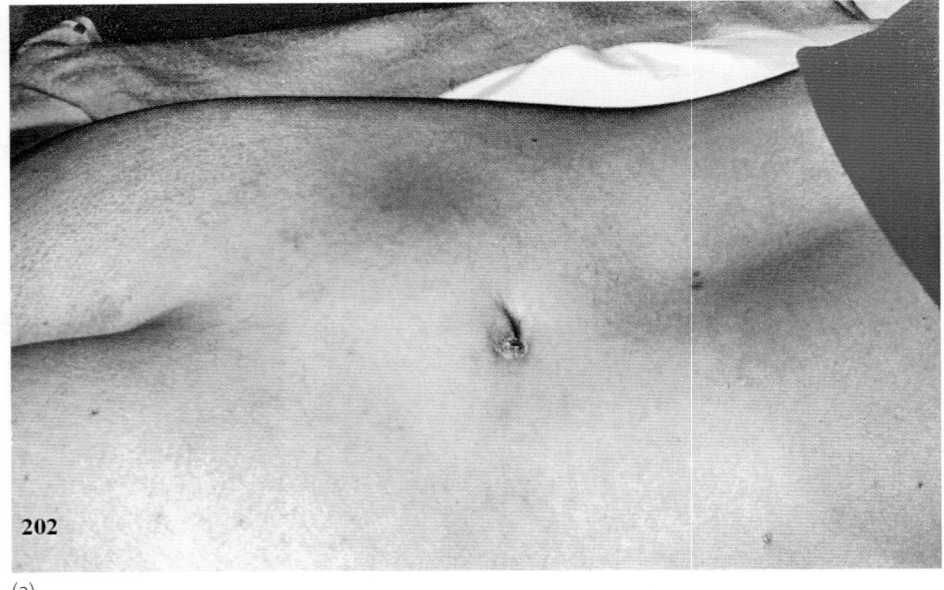

(a)

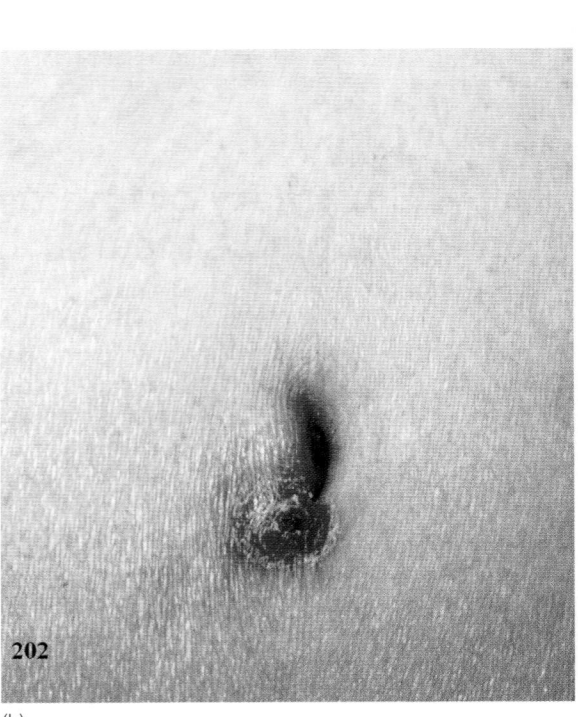

(b)

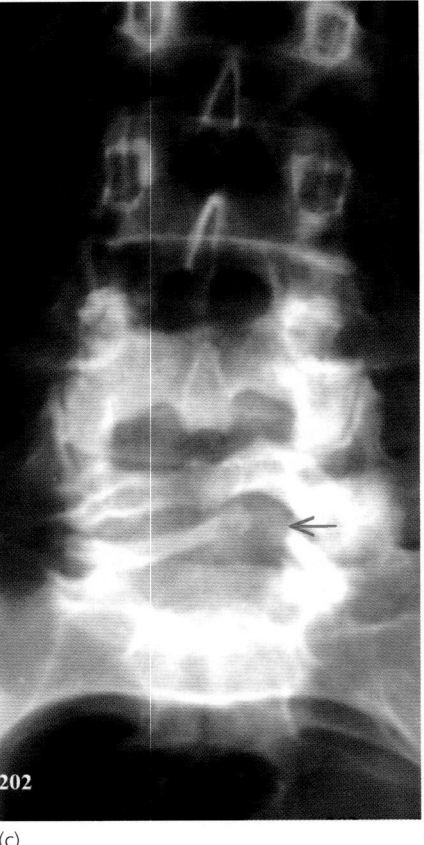

(c)

Fig. 8.25 (a) View of patient's back with dermal sinus tract, presenting as a dimple at L4–5. (b) Close-up view of dimple, with raised cystic mass and punctum. (c) Anteroposterior (AP) radiograph of the same patient, with spina bifida at S1, and associated distortion of L5.

8.6 Conclusions

This chapter has described only some of the many and varied diseases of the spine and their surgical treatment, which may interfere with the successful establishment of epidural block. The use of epidurograms may help to advance our knowledge of the pathological processes involved and how best to overcome them. In the meantime, patients with significant back problems can present a rare challenge, but the results are often highly beneficial and rewarding. However, it does appear that even minor degrees of scoliosis, of which the patient may be unaware, can lead to unsatisfactory blocks far more often than is recognized.

REFERENCES

1 Campbell DC (2000) Musculoskeletal Disorders. In *Textbook of Obstetric Anesthesia*, editors Birnbach DJ, Gatt SP, Datta S. Churchill Livingstone, Philadelphia, pp. 617–629.

2 Tolo VT (1989) Surgical treatment of adult adolescent idiopathic scoliosis. *Instructional Course Lectures*; 38:143–146.

3 Schachner SM, Abram SE (1982) Use of two epidural catheters to provide analgesia of unblocked segments in a patient with lumbar disc disease. *Anesthesiology*; 56:150–151.

4 Moran DH, Johnson MD (1990) Continuous spinal anesthesia with combined hyperbaric and isobaric bupivacaine in a patient with scoliosis. *Anesthesia and Analgesia*; 70:445–447.

5 Pascoe HE, Jennings GS, Marx GF (1993) Successful spinal anesthesia after inadequate epidural block in a parturient with prior surgical correction of scoliosis. *Regional Anesthesia*; 18:191–192.

6 Daley MD, Rolbin SH, Hew EM, Morningstar BA, Stewart JA (1990) Epidural anesthesia for obstetrics after spinal surgery. *Regional Anesthesia*; 15:280–284.

7 Lee YJ, Bundschu RH, Moffat EC (1995) Unintentional subdural block during labor epidural in a parturient with prior Harrington rod insertion for scoliosis. *Regional Anesthesia*; 20:159–162.

8 Hu SS, Tribus CB, Diab M, Ghanayem AJ (2008) Spondylolisthesis and spondylolysis. *Instructional Course Lectures*; 57:431–435.

9 Kumar R, Guinto FC Jr, Madewell JE (1988) The vertebral body: Radiographic configurations in various congenital and acquired disorders. *Radiographics*; 8:455–485.

10 McGrady EM, Davis AG (1988) Spina bifida occulta and epidural anaesthesia. *Anaesthesia*; 43:857–859.

11 Davies PRF, Loach AB (1996) Spinal anaesthesia and spina-bifida occulta. *Anaesthesia*; 51:1158–1160.

12 Page LK (1985) Occult spinal dysraphism and related disorders. In *Neurosurgery*, editors Wilkins RH, Rengachary SS. McGraw-Hill, New York, pp. 259–265.

13 Altamimi Y, Pavy TJ (2006) Epidural analgesia for labour in a patient with a neural tube defect. *Anaesthesia and Intensive Care*; 34:816–819.

14 Albano JP, Shannon SG, Alem NM, Mason KT (1996) Injury risk for research subjects with spina bifida occulta in a repeated impact study: a case review. *Aviation, Space and Environmental Medicine*; 67:767–769.

15 Collier CB (2010) The intradural space: the fourth place to go astray during attempted epidural block. *International Journal of Obstetric Anesthesia*; 19:133–141.

16 Samuel M, Boddy SA (2004) Is spina bifida occulta associated with lower urinary tract dysfunction in children? *Journal of Urology*; 171:2644–2666.

17 Sairyo K, Goel VK, Vadapalli S (2006) Biomechanical comparison of lumbar spine with or without spina bifida occulta. A finite element analysis. *Spinal Cord*; 44:440–4446.

CHAPTER 9
AN ASSESSMENT OF EPIDURAL CATHETERS: THE ROLE OF EPIDUROGRAMS

9.1 Introduction

Our epidurogram study has provided a unique opportunity to assess the many types of epidural catheter that were available at the time (Table 9.1). On various occasions, the radiographic examinations were combined with our published clinical studies on the functioning of the catheters in mainly obstetric practice.[1,2] We hoped to be able to state the ideal properties required for an epidural catheter, particularly with regard to catheter rigidity and the number of eyes and their positioning. Our previous conclusions included recommending against the use of terminal hole catheters in obstetric patients because of an unacceptably high incidence of unsatisfactory blocks in the congested epidural space of term pregnancy.[2] However, this recommendation now seems only to apply to the older, more rigid, types of catheter.

● **Table 9.1** Summary of catheter usage in 178 patients (final insertion only, if more than one catheter was used)

CATHETER TYPE	n
Portex 17 gauge three lateral eyes	86
Portex 17 gauge three closer eyes	43
Arrow 19 gauge terminal hole	22
Portex 17 gauge terminal hole	4
Portex 19 gauge three lateral eyes	4
Mallinckrodt 20 gauge terminal hole	2
Becton Dickinson 20 gauge terminal hole	2
CSE Portex (combined spinal epidural) 17 gauge three lateral eyes	15

9.2 Catheter rigidity

Initially, over the first 10 years or so of this work, the only catheters available were fairly rigid in construction, leading to a high incidence of significant paraesthesiae (23%) and blood vessel perforation (6%) during insertion.[2] Catheters with softer flexible tips were then introduced by some manufacturers, with occasional unforeseen results (Fig. 9.1).

The current trend of incorporating coiled wire within the polyurethane or nylon of the catheter wall has produced softer, more flexible catheters, with a reduced incidence and severity of paraesthesiae (3–5%), as well as a lessened risk of vascular damage (1%).[3] However, many anaesthetists, particularly those in training, report difficulty with inserting soft catheters through epidural needles, even when a

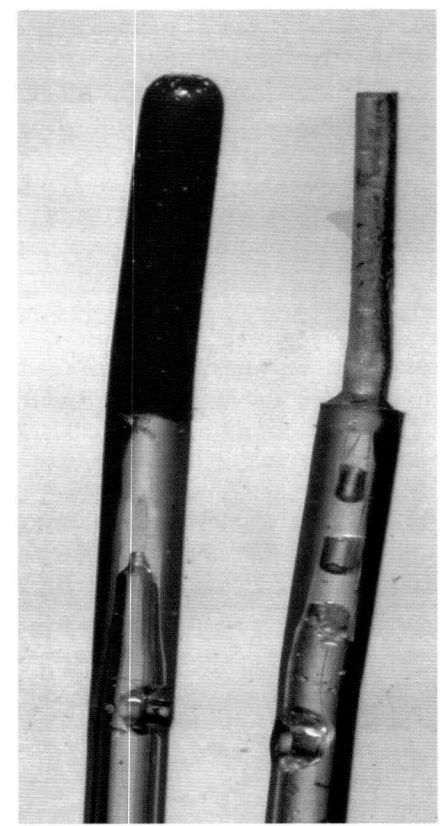

● **Fig. 9.1** Intact Braun flexible tip catheter on the left, with absent tip on the right, following removal from patient.

threading assistance device is used, and the use of more rigid catheters persists despite the obvious advantages of the softer types. In addition, the softer catheters are often more difficult to extract at the end of the procedure.

9.3 How many holes/eyes are enough?

There have also been changes in the number and positioning of the holes or eyes that are incorporated into the catheter design.[4] The first prepackaged epidural catheters were simply plain tubes, open at each end, but the distal opening could be traumatic to structures in the epidural space, and this was later rounded off. Other manufacturers closed off the distal end and incorporated one, two, three, six, even 12 or more lateral openings in their catheters, often with little scientific data to support the changes. Three lateral holes appeared to be the most popular end result, but where to site them became a contentious matter, once manufacturing difficulties had been overcome. We trialled three different models of Portex catheter (Portex Ltd, Ashford, Kent, UK) with the standard eyes at 6/10/14 mm from the tip, the closer-eye at 2/3/4 mm, and an intermediate model at 4/6/8 mm (Fig. 9.2), with little detectable difference in function. To date, we have been unable to demonstrate any improved safety from having the eyes moved closer together.

9.3.1 Blocked catheter eyes

Epidural catheters with three lateral eyes are prone to blockage by blood clot, particularly in obstetric patients and after prolonged insertion.[4] Occasionally, catheters will have to be replaced when clot in the lumen, or in all three eyes, makes injection impossible. Blockage of one or two eyes may be associated with inadequate block, as restricted flow and distribution of local anaesthetic may occur through the patent eyes, which are of far smaller cross-sectional area than the typical terminal hole.

FAILED CAESAREAN SECTION BLOCK

A 31-year-old patient in labour had a catheter with three lateral eyes (Portex) inserted at L3–4 to a depth of 3 cm within the epidural space, without incident. Although the upper level of the block reached T9 bilaterally, there was persistent failure to block any sacral roots despite repeated doses of local anaesthetic. When an emergency caesarean section became necessary, top-up of the block with 20 mL lidocaine 2% with adrenaline appeared to block the sacral roots, and extend upwards to T4 bilaterally when tested with pin-prick. Surgery commenced and was satisfactory until the uterus was exteriorized immediately following delivery, when severe lower abdominal pain developed at the T12 level, predominantly on the right side. General anaesthesia was induced to treat the pain. A postoperative infusion patient-controlled epidural analgesia (PCEA) of bupivacaine 0.125% with fentanyl produced only a reasonable level of analgesia and was discontinued after 4 h.

Epidurogram findings: maldistribution of contrast
Screening of the epidurogram, on the following day, revealed the catheter tip at L2–3 in the midline, pointing cephalad. There was considerable resistance to contrast injection, with the initial spread being fairly uniform between L2 and L4. Above this, the contrast extended to T11 as two lateral columns, with reduced midline spread. There was a large filling defect (arrowed, Fig. 9.3a)

● **Fig. 9.2** The three models of Portex epidural catheter used in this work, with variable eye spacings (from left to right): the closer eye, intermediate and standard catheters.

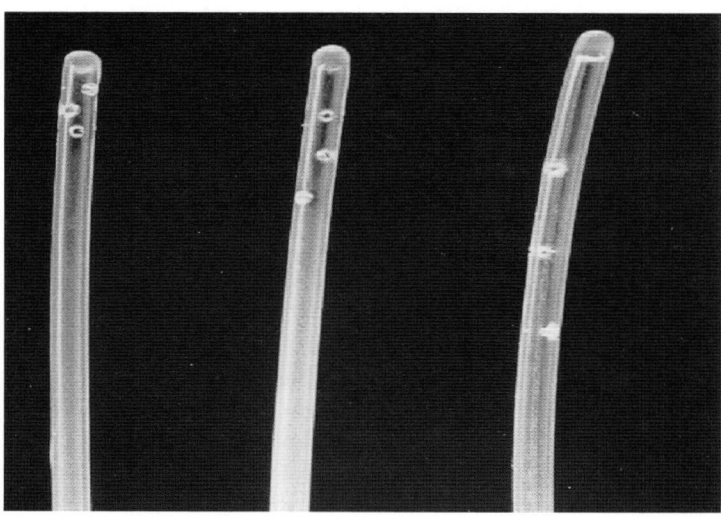

● **Fig. 9.3** (a) Anteroposterior (AP) epidurogram following failed block for caesarean section. There is a large, predominantly right-sided, filling defect at L1–2 (arrowed). (b) Lateral epidurogram showing attenuation of the posterior column of contrast (between the arrows) at the level of the filling defect.

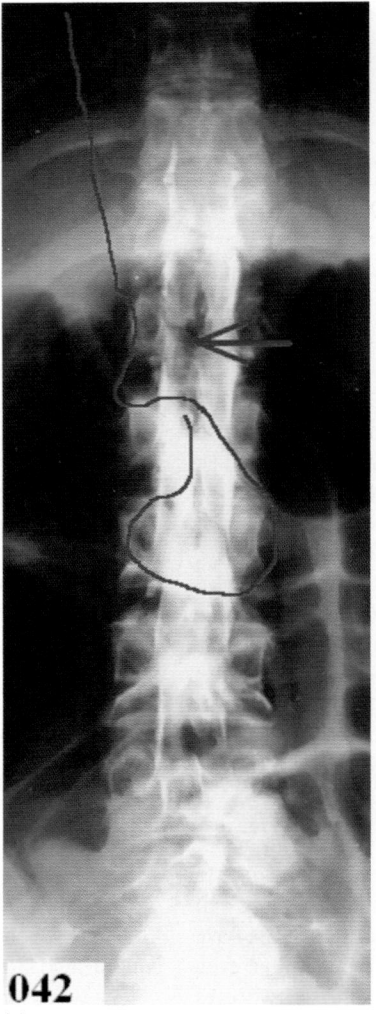

(a)

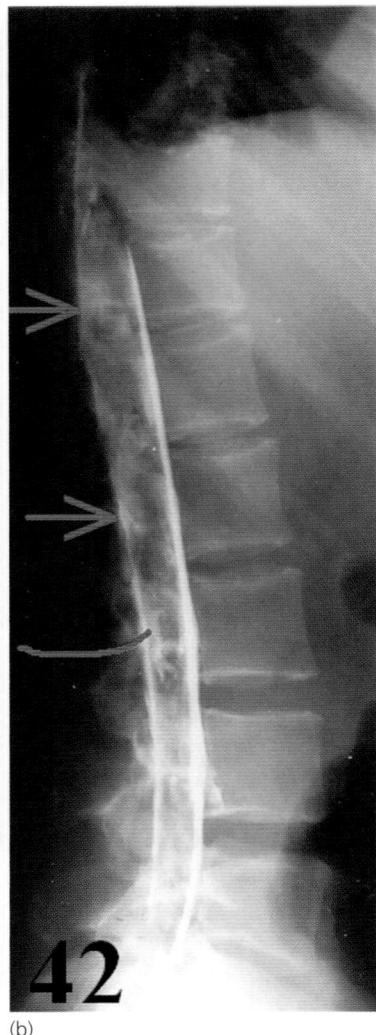

(b)

predominantly to the right of the midline at L1–2, which appears to correspond with the clinically unblocked areas. The foraminal contrast escape was sparse above L3. In the lateral view (Fig. 9.3b) there is a fairly uniform spread of contrast across the epidural space, with a marked anterior column, but an attenuated posterior column between T12 and L2 (arrowed), at the site of the filling defect.

Catheter examination: **single patent eye**

Following removal of the epidural catheter, it was subjected to close examination, as part of our study of 2000 consecutive used catheters.[4] Saline flushed through the catheter met with considerable resistance, and slowly exited through the proximal eye only, when considerable injection pressure was applied. Microscopic examination revealed the presence of some debris completely blocking the lumen of the catheter between the proximal and middle eyes.

Aspiration of saline through the catheter caused the debris to move more proximally, where it was photographed (Fig. 9.3c) and then excised. The nature of the hard white material could not be ascertained, but it was presumed to be a fragment of nylon 'swarf' remaining after the eye-drilling process in manufacture. The resulting obstruction may have accounted for the contrast maldistribution and the unsatisfactory block as, almost certainly, only one small catheter eye was patent within the epidural space.

9.3.2 Terminal hole catheters

In a study comparing lateral eye with terminal hole catheters in obstetric practice, using the older, more rigid type catheters, we found that the incidence of unsatisfactory blocks with

● **Fig. 9.3** (Continued) (c) The blocked catheter, with obstructive debris or 'swarf' (arrowed).

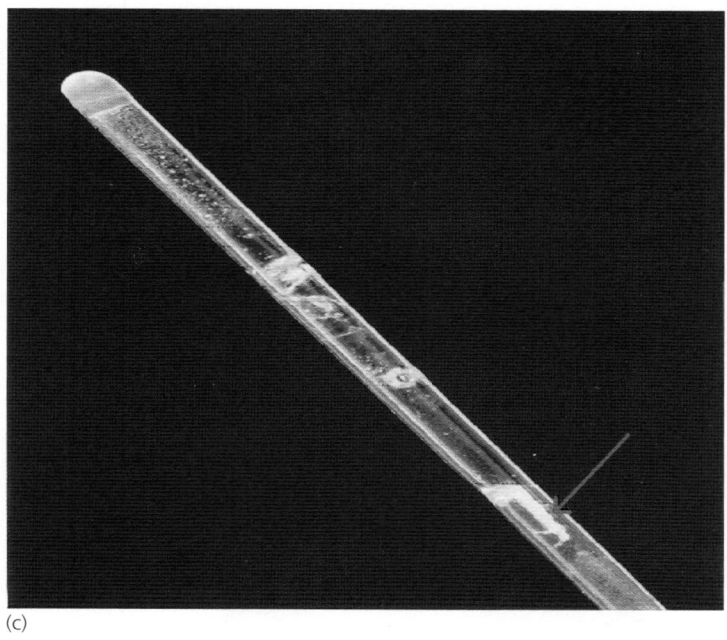

(c)

the latter was unacceptably high (32%), when compared with lateral eyes (12%), with unilateral and patchy missed segment block comprising the majority of failures.[2] This was attributed to the poor lateral spread of injected solutions exiting the terminal hole, as these solutions tend to form a single unidirectional stream away from the tip, whereas with lateral eyes there are usually three streams separated by arcs of 120° and a length of a few millimetres.[4] However, this may be a rather simplistic explanation, as in the crowded lumbar epidural space of term pregnancy, the tip of a catheter is likely to be surrounded by epidural fat and blood vessels, so that no streams of emerging solution usually arise, merely a collection of trickling fluid. Furthermore, laboratory studies have shown that, using moderate injection pressures, the proximal eye of a lateral eye catheter is the main conduit for fluid to exit, with the other eyes being largely redundant.[4] Whatever the mechanism, our poor results led us to recommend against using terminal eye catheters, at least in obstetrics.

When a soft flexible wire-coil catheter first became available we requested that the manufacturer (Arrow International, Reading, PA, USA) produce a lateral eye model, but this was technically difficult at that time, although now available (Portex). We started using the flexible (Arrow) catheter and found the terminal hole now to be satisfactory, and a recent study by Spiegel et al.[3] has confirmed our findings that there were no differences in the initial analgesia success rate, complications or labour analgesia between terminal hole and lateral eye flexible catheters. The authors attribute the success of the new catheters to their ability to coil in the epidural space

and stay near the midline, rather than heading laterally towards the intervertebral foramina, with the chance of catheter escape.

9.4 Modified catheter lumen – the 'Ribbed' catheter

The Becton Dickinson (Franklin Lakes, NJ, USA) Perisafe 'ribbed catheter' was designed with a unique irregular lumen (Fig. 9.4), in an attempt to overcome the problem of

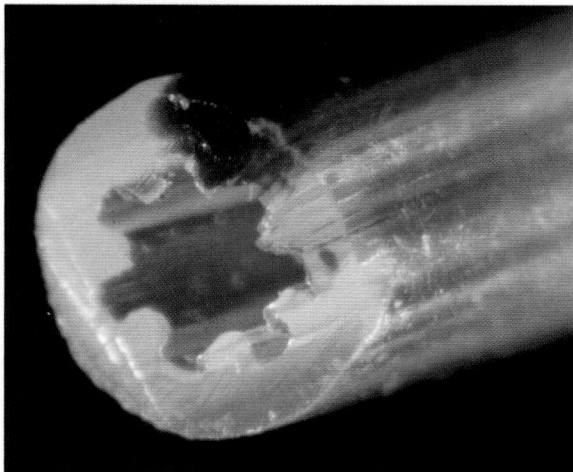

● **Fig. 9.4** A view of the distal end of a 'ribbed' Perisafe catheter (Becton Dickinson) showing the unique irregular lumen.

soft catheters kinking and obstructing within the epidural space. We used such a catheter in 12 patients with limited success, as catheter obstruction was a recurring feature. All 12 catheters felt fairly rigid on insertion. Epidurograms on two of these patients with failed blocks demonstrated that the catheters were deviated laterally: out through an intervertebral foramen in one (Fig. 9.5) and to the right lateral border of the epidural space in the other (Fig. 9.6), with a persistent unilateral block developing. It seems likely that these initially rigid catheters developed increased compliance at body temperature, and were then more likely to become kinked and obstructed. In five of the 12 patients, the catheter had to be replaced. No contrast could be injected through those kinked catheters that were left *in situ*.

This particular type of catheter gained little popularity as it appeared to combine two adverse properties: the early rigidity and the later compressibility.

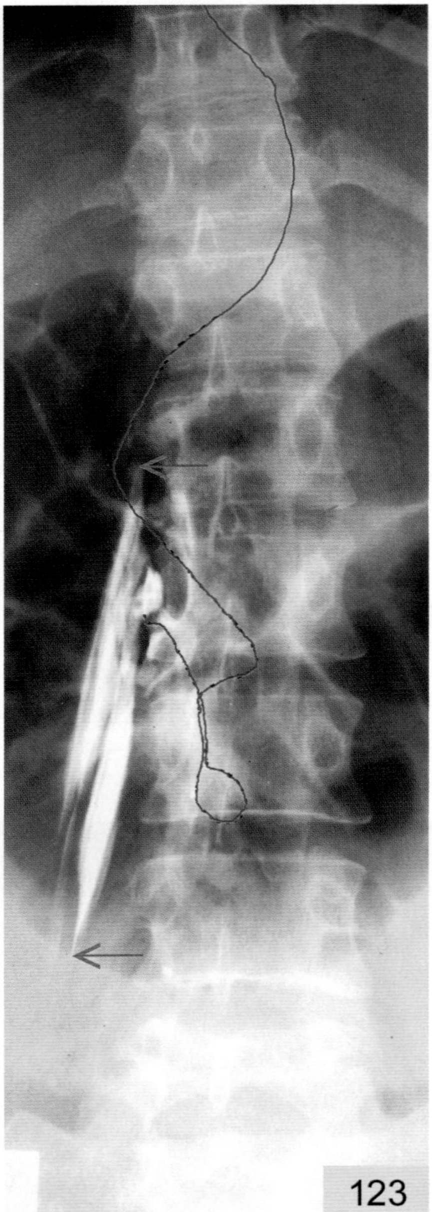

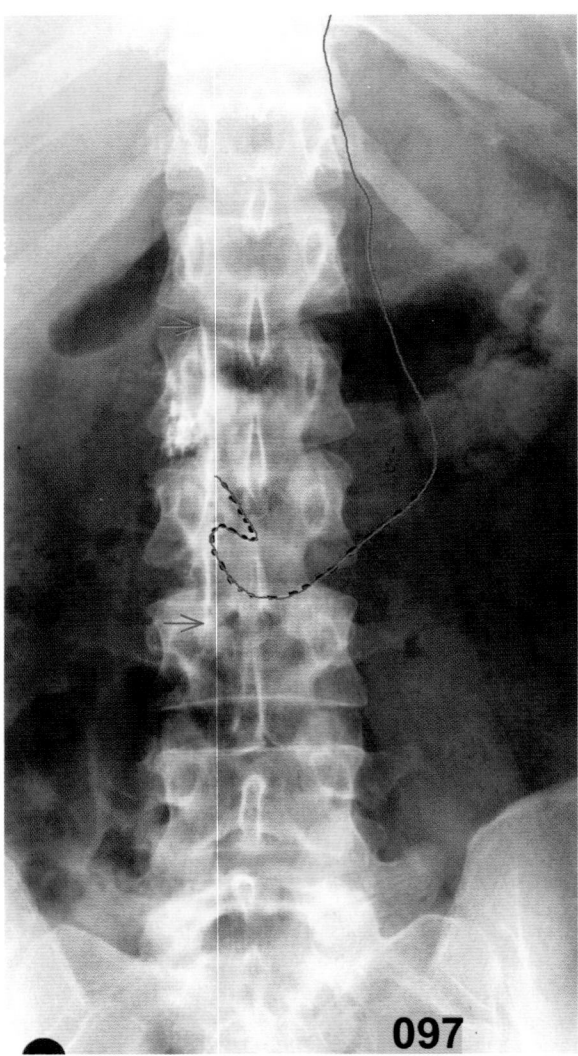

● **Fig. 9.5** Anteroposterior (AP) epidurogram showing a mild degree of scoliosis with a ribbed Perisafe catheter inserted at L2–3 to the right of the midline, deviating laterally and escaping through the L2–3 foramen, and contrast collecting anterior to the psoas muscle (arrowed).

● **Fig. 9.6** Anteroposterior (AP) epidurogram showing a Perisafe ribbed catheter inserted at L3–4 in the midline, and running laterally to the right. Contrast injection (7 mL) flowed into a narrow right lateral epidural column between L2 and L4 (arrowed) with transforaminal spill only at the L2–3 foramen.

9.5 Direction of the catheter tip following epidural insertion

Usubiaga et al. in 1970 were among the first to use radiographic studies to follow the path of epidural catheters and relate the positioning of the catheter tip to the efficiency of the neuraxial block.[5] More recently, Hogan used computed tomography (CT) imaging to detect catheter tip position and relate it to the functioning of the prior epidural block, but they could not assess the direction in which the catheter tip was pointing.[6]

In our series of 178 patients (193 catheters in situ at the time of radiography) the position of the catheter tip could only be determined in 180 instances.

9.5.1 Attempted direction of insertion

The vast majority of the 176 catheters had been inserted using a midline approach with the bevel of the Tuohy needle pointing upwards (in a cephalad direction). Two catheters were inserted through a lateral-pointing bevel (see section 9.5.2.1) and two with a downwards (caudal) direction, once intentionally and once in error.

9.5.2 Final position of the catheter tip

Of the 176 epidural catheters that had been inserted in a cephalad direction, 143 (81%) followed this direction with 17 (10%) running predominantly caudally (Fig. 9.7). The remaining 16 (9%) catheters ran laterally, with 10 escaping

143 (81%) cephalad

176 catheters directed cephalad → 16 (9%) lateral → 10 (6%) escaped, 6 (3%) lateral

17 (10%) caudad

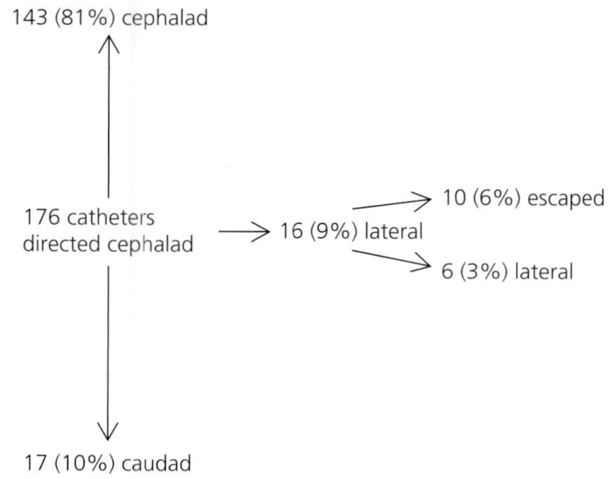

Fig. 9.7 Direction of catheter travel.

through an intervertebral foramen and six remaining in a lateral recess of the epidural space.

The most likely cause of caudal displacement was found to be an obstruction within the epidural space, usually a septum or postsurgical adhesions. Use of a 'softer' catheter in these patients may have predisposed them to displacement. Catheters sited outside the epidural space, such as those in the subarachnoid intradural or subdural spaces, or paravertebral space, appeared to run unconstrained in all directions.

9.5.2.1 Lateral catheter placement

We only have epidurograms on two patients with epidural catheters deliberately inserted through laterally directed bevels, but it seems likely, on clinical grounds at least, that epidural catheters, especially the more rigid ones, inserted in this direction are more likely to be associated with failed blocks for obstetrics or general surgery than ones directed cranially. The insertion of Tuohy needles with lateral-pointing bevels became popular many years ago for two reasons. First, to deliberately produce a predominantly unilateral block, mostly for surgery on one lower limb, and second, based on the rather dubious theory that the bundles of collagen fibres that form the dura ran parallel to the vertebral column and if accidental dural puncture did occur, then the size of the dural hole would be minimized. We now recognize that the collagen fibres run in all directions,[7] so that the practice of bevel rotation should cease unless specifically indicated to produce a unilateral block, particularly for day surgery.

A laterally directed catheter, of insufficient length to escape through an intervertebral foramen, may be positioned with its tip in a lateral recess of the epidural space (as in Fig. 9.6). This positioning does not appear conducive to effective bilateral spread of local anaesthetic, especially if a terminal hole or closer-eye is in use, with restricted spread of injectate away from the catheter tip.

CASE HISTORY 9.2:
PREDOMINANTLY UNILATERAL BLOCK

A closer-eye catheter (Portex) was inserted in a labouring patient at L3–4 with the Tuohy needle bevel accidentally rotated to the left. A 4 cm length of catheter was introduced into the epidural space. Even after repeated boluses of 0.375% bupivacaine, to a total dose of 42 mL, block on the right side was poor and patchy, and never above T12, while the left side was blocked to T7.

Epidurogram findings: maldistribution of contrast
On AP screening the following day the catheter tip was noted to be laterally placed to the left at the level of the L3–4 interspace. The left side of the main body of contrast filled first and was of greater density than the

127

right. The AP view (Fig. 9.8a) shows the restricted spread of contrast from L1–5, with bilateral foraminal spill, which was more marked and extensive on the left. In the lateral view (Fig. 9.8b), contrast appears to be uniformly spread across the epidural space. The epidurogram did suggest some degree of obstruction caused by a midline septum, but it is difficult to assess how much of the poor block and uneven distribution of contrast resulted from obstructive factors, rather than an aberrant catheter tip.

Following the epidurogram the epidural catheter was cautiously removed and inspected. A fixed curve of the distal 5 cm of catheter through 90° to the left was observed.

9.5.2.2 Caudal catheter placement

A closer look at the 17 cases where the cephalad-directed catheters had been diverted caudally revealed that four were in the subarachnoid, subdural or intradural spaces.

Of the 13 catheters displaced caudally within the epidural space, 10 were the older more rigid type (7.1% of these catheters), with the remaining three being the current softer catheters (with 13.6% of these being displaced).

Clinically, the use of the 13 caudally pointing catheters positioned in the epidural space provided satisfactory blocks in only three cases, with most of the blocks being too low or patchy. In assessing this high incidence of failures,

● **Fig. 9.8**
(a) Anteroposterior (AP) epidurogram through a laterally placed catheter tip (closer eye). Contrast is seen from L1 to L5, more densely on the left, following a persistent left unilateral block. Transforaminal spill of contrast (arrowed) is also far more prolific on the left. (b) Lateral epidurogram, showing a fairly uniform spread of contrast across the epidural space from T12 to L5 (arrowed). The combined views suggest the presence of a midline septum associated with lateral placement of the catheter tip.

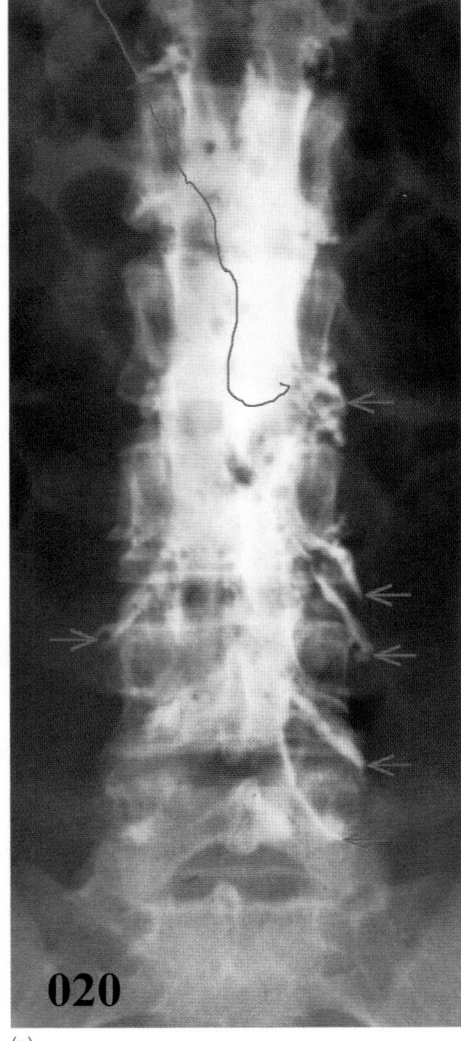

(a)

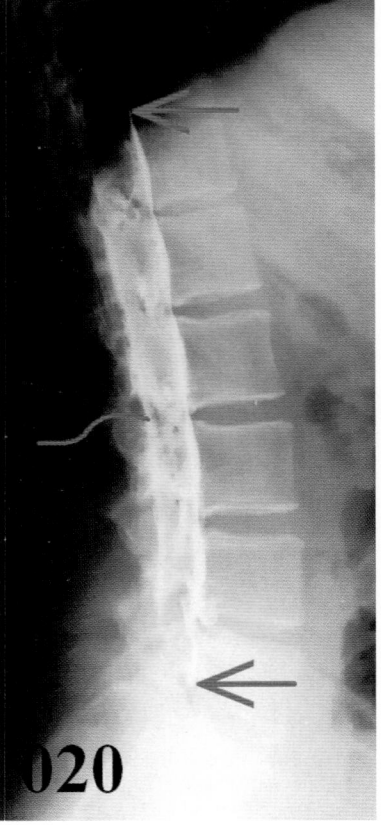

(b)

it should not be forgotten that most of the epidurograms in this series were performed to investigate failed or inadequate blocks.

Some of these 17 cases with caudally positioned catheters are now described:

1 **Catheter displaced by septum:** this case, featuring a transverse septum, has already been described in detail (Fig. 7.9a, p.96) but the plain radiograph (Fig. 9.9) clearly shows the caudal direction of the catheter. The block was too low, not spreading above T10.

2 **Catheter in the subarachnoid, subdural or intradural space:** while about 90% of catheters directed cephalad in the epidural space tended to run in that direction, catheters misplaced outside the epidural space seemed not to be so constrained. Of the three cases of subdural block studied, the catheter turned caudally in one (Fig. 5.3a, p.46). Similarly, in at least two of the 10 cases of intradural block the catheter ran caudally (Fig. 5.5a, p.50, and Fig. 5.9a, p.55) although the incidence may have been higher as the catheter tip was often impossible to visualize because of the dense collection of contrast that characterizes this complication.

3 **Catheter displaced without obvious obstruction:** the caudal positioning of a catheter tip did not always result in an inadequate block, as the next case, using a softer catheter, illustrates (Case History 9.3).

CASE HISTORY 9.3:
SATISFACTORY BLOCK

A 19-gauge lateral eye catheter (Portex) was inserted uneventfully at L2–3 in a cephalad direction in a 40-year-old patient. Satisfactory block for abdominal hysterectomy ensued.

Epidurogram findings: limited foraminal contrast spill

Fluoroscopic screening revealed the catheter to be running caudally, with the tip at L3, well to the right of the midline. The initial contrast flowed predominantly to the left side in a distinct column from T10 to L4, with limited foraminal contrast escape. A right-sided column appeared next, and the final appearance (Fig. 9.10a) was fairly symmetrical, but with only a small volume of foraminal spill at L3–4 bilaterally. The lateral view (Fig. 9.10b) shows patchy contrast across the width of the epidural space, with the posterior column being predominant and only an attenuated anterior column above L2.

With the early contrast flow being largely unilateral, and no contrast appearing below L4, there may be some evidence of a septum partly obstructing the flow of epidural solutions, or the picture may simply have resulted from the catheter tip not being in an ideal position. However, the block was satisfactory, so that it appears that more work is required to define the ideal positioning of the epidural catheter tip.

In summary, caudal displacement of catheters appears to be more common in the presence of a septum or other obstruction, following insertion outside the epidural space and with the use of more flexible, narrow-gauge catheters. It is perhaps not unexpected that these softer catheters could be more easily displaced by obstructions in their path.

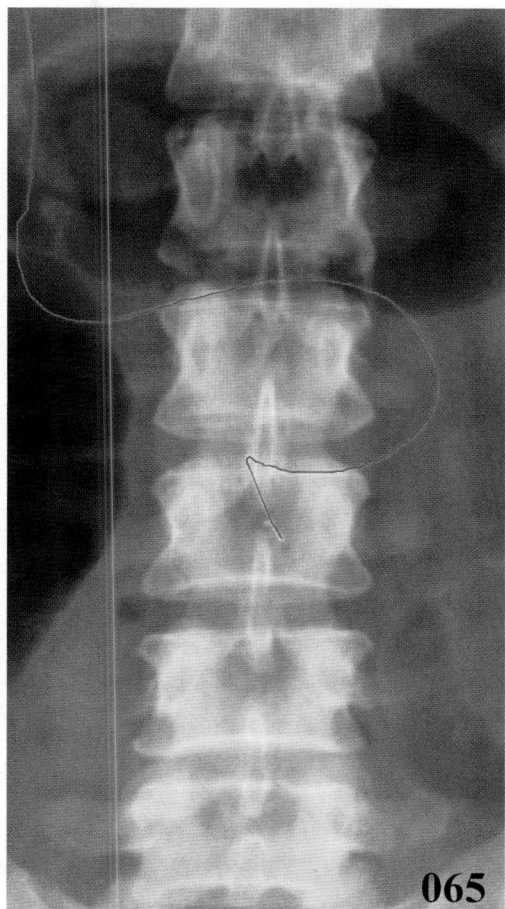

065

● **Fig. 9.9** Anteroposterior (AP) radiograph of thoracolumbar spine showing a radio-opaque 19 gauge flexible-tip catheter (Arrow) running caudally, despite cephalad insertion (see Fig. 7.9a, p.96).

● **Fig. 9.10** (a) Anteroposterior (AP) epidurogram revealing a 19 gauge catheter (Portex) running caudally, despite cephalad insertion, with fairly extensive vertical spread of contrast from T10 to L4 (arrowed) but only minimal transforaminal spill at L3–4, following a successful block. (b) Lateral epidurogram showing the caudal direction of the catheter, with fairly extensive and uniform spread of contrast (arrowed) but with an attenuated anterior column above L2.

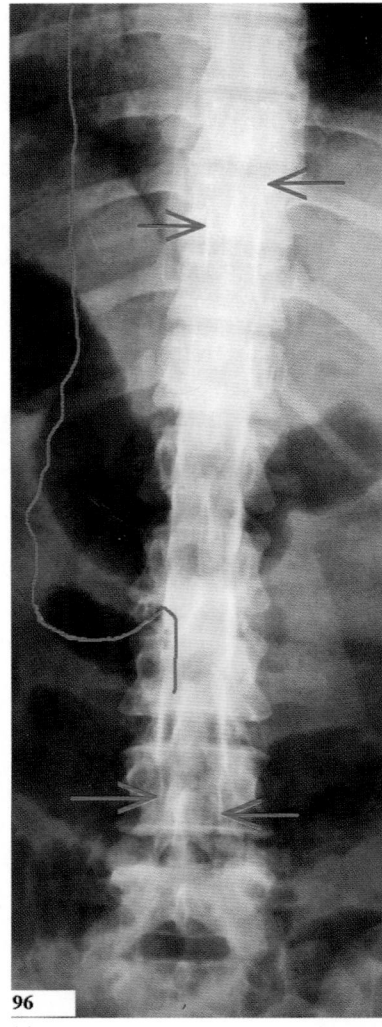

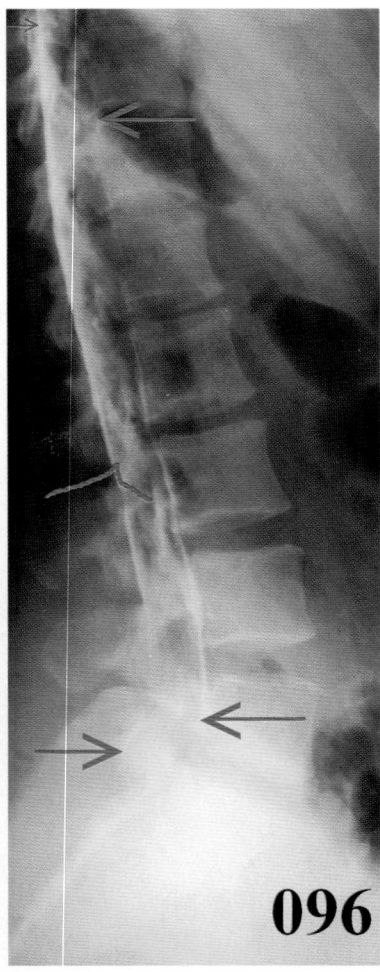

(a)　　　　　　　　　(b)

9.6 Conclusion

The introduction of disposable epidural catheters in 1962 led to explosive growth in the popularity of epidural block. Both the design of catheters and the materials used in their construction have slowly improved over the past few decades. Softer catheters appear to be ideal, in terms of reduced trauma to nervous tissue and blood vessels, although they may be more difficult to insert, particularly for the inexperienced. They are also more likely to be displaced from their intended location in the midline of the epidural space pointing cephalad, as is desirable in most situations. The number of catheter eyes or their spacing at the catheter tip appears to be of no great significance if softer catheters are used.

REFERENCES

1 Collier CB, Gatt SP (1993) A new epidural catheter. Closer eyes for safety? *Anaesthesia*; 48:803–806.

2 Collier CB, Gatt SP (1994) Epidural catheters for obstetrics; terminal hole or lateral eyes? *Regional Anesthesia*; 19:378–385.

3 Spiegel JE, Vasudevan A, Li Y, Hess PE (2009) A randomised prospective study comparing two flexible epidural catheters for labour analgesia. *British Journal of Anaesthesia*; 103: 400–405.

4 Collier CB (1994) *Some Complications of Epidural Block.* Doctor of Medicine Thesis. University of New South Wales, Sydney, Australia.

5 Usubiaga JE, dos Reis A Jr, Usubiaga LE (1970) Epidural misplacement of catheters and mechanisms of unilateral blockade. *Anesthesiology*; 32:158–161.

6 Hogan QH (1999) Epidural catheter tip position and distribution of injectate evaluated by computed tomography. *Anesthesiology*; 90: 964–970.

7 Reina MA, Casasola ODL, Lopez A, De Andres JA, Mora M, Fernandez A (2002) The origin of the spinal subdural space: Ultrastructure findings. *Anesthesia and Analgesia*; 94:991–995.

CHAPTER 10
CONCLUSIONS

The illustrations in this book provide an array of only a small proportion of the very diverse images that have appeared following contrast injection through epidural catheters on almost 180 instances. Much more work remains to be done, particularly in regard to the septum, which seems to play a pivotal role in the majority of cases of failed or inadequate epidural block.

In most situations, there has been significant correlation between the extent of the neuraxial block and the subsequent epidurogram findings. Where the two have been at variance, the use of a greater volume of contrast may often have clarified the situation. However, at the start of this work there was still concern about the possible toxicity of the available contrast media, and we elected to use a standard 10–13 mL dose (depending on body weight) to enable us to compare the degree of filling of the epidural space between patients. This may have hampered the interpretation of some of the radiographs, and doses of up to 20 mL may be advantageous, as long as subarachnoid injection has been excluded.

No correlation was evident in three particular obstetric patients, where repeated epidural block had been unsatisfactory, yet a normal distribution of contrast was later revealed by epidurography. Two of these patients were regular and long-term intravenous heroin users, and it is interesting to speculate whether there is a change in receptor susceptibility to local anaesthetic blockade in the addicted patient. It has been proposed that, following opiate withdrawal, hyperalgesia results from activation of a specific descending modulatory system, mediated partly by spinal cord κ and α-2 adrenergic receptors, and attenuated by clonidine.[1] This effect may be more likely following epidural than subarachnoid block and may account for the apparent failure of correctly sited epidural local anaesthetic in opioid-dependent patients.[2] The third patient suffered quite marked Ehlers–Danlos syndrome (Hypermobility Type III) with paper-thin skin and hypermobile joints. Initial epidural needle insertion resulted in dural puncture, which appeared to be related to a highly attenuated ligamentum flavum. A cautious repeat epidural block in an adjoining interspace produced very patchy epidural analgesia for labour, as has been reported in some patients with Ehlers–Danlos syndrome.[3] The epidurogram showed normal contrast spread. There is also the extremely rare possibility of local anaesthetic resistance, where correctly placed blocks repeatedly fail, due to local anaesthetic receptor mutations and anomalies of the sodium channels.[4] A genetic variation in the amino acid sequence within these channels may reduce the efficiency of the receptor sites. While these unusual types of block failure are very interesting, it must not be forgotten that the vast majority of block failures result from poor operator technique or an anatomical anomaly.

We have seen that the use of epidurograms may be useful in diagnosing unusual or potentially life-threatening complications of epidural block, although this may be of little benefit to the patient involved. Some of the mechanisms responsible for the occasional failure of epidural block, whether total or partial, have been elucidated. This knowledge may be of value in improving the operator's standard of practice and efficiency, as well as providing some explanation and reassurance regarding future blocks to an anxious and possibly aggrieved patient. We would encourage our colleagues to investigate at least some of their own failed or complicated blocks, and personally inject the contrast during the screening procedure. The investigation takes only a few minutes, and the results can be most intriguing and enlightening.

To summarize our main conclusions, in teaching hospital practice, with many inexperienced operators, the commonest cause of epidural failure is that the epidural catheter is not in the epidural space. If the catheter has been inserted correctly then the commonest cause of failure or inadequacy is the presence of a midline or transverse septum, which may be difficult to overcome. Less commonly the catheter tip may escape from the epidural space through an intervertebral foramen, and the incidence of this may possibly be reduced by using softer catheters and only inserting 2–3 cm into the space. Partial withdrawal of the catheter and redosing may remedy the situation in about 50% of cases. Finally, the presence of even mild degrees of scoliosis, of which the patient is often unaware, seems to be associated with unilateral or patchy blocks, particularly when low-dose epidural solutions are used in labour.

It does appear as if the current generation of softer and more flexible catheters, incorporating coiled wire, are resulting in improved results in terms of block efficiency and reduced failure rate, while having a lower incidence of nerve and blood vessel trauma on insertion. Their only drawbacks appear to be increased difficulty of catheter insertion and removal, particularly for the inexperienced, and the occasional problem arising from the displacement of these softer catheters away from their intended cephalad positioning within the epidural space. The number and positioning of the catheter holes or eyes does not seem to be particularly important with these newer catheters.

Many workers still believe that the most consistently reliable epidural blocks result from injection through the wide bore of the epidural needle itself, rather than a catheter. Whatever equipment is used, attention to the minor details of epidural technique, as well as simple but accurate assessment of the resulting block, and remedial measures where required, are essential for success.

REFERENCES

1 Sood V, Robinson DA, Suri I (2009) Difficult intubation during rapid sequence induction in a parturient with Ehlers–Danlos syndrome, hypermobility type. *International Journal of Obstetric Anesthesia*; 18:408–412.

2 Aviles J, Barbaro NM, Drasner K (1993) Pharmacology of descending hyperalgesia: Evidence for involvement of spinal cord kappa and alpha-adrenergic receptors. *Anesthesiology*; 79(Suppl):A906.

3 Golomb E, Langerman L, Benita S (1993) Discrepancy between the development of tolerance to bupivacaine in extradural and spinal anaesthesia in rabbits. *British Journal of Anaesthesia*; 71:450–452.

4 Kavlock R, Ting PH (2004) Local anesthetic resistance in a pregnant patient with lumbosacral plexopathy. *BMC Anesthesiology*; 4:1; http//www.biomedcentral.com/bmcanesthesiol/ (accessed 9/5/11).

Index

Note: page numbers in **bold** refer to diagrams, page numbers in *italics* refer to information contained in tables.

137